THE
SPIRITUAL
HEALING
HANDBOOK

How to develop your healing powers and
increase your spiritual awareness

JACK & JAN ANGELO

PIATKUS

TO

the indigenous peoples who have kept the sacred at the
heart of their communities

First published as *Sacred Healing* in 2001 by Piatkus Books

This edition published in 2007

A CIP catalogue record for this book
is available from the British Library

ISBN 978-0-7499-2825-4

Data manipulation by
4word Ltd, Bristol
Printed and bound in
Great Britain by MPG Books,
Bodmin, Cornwall

Piatkus Books
An imprint of
Little, Brown Book Group
100 Victoria Embankment
London EC4Y 0DY

An Hachette Livre UK Company

www.piatkus.co.uk

Contents

The Action Points

Acknowledgements

We would like to thank all those who have shared their journeys with us.

The case histories have been chosen to illustrate specific teaching points. Names and situations have been changed to protect privacy and preserve confidentiality.

We would also like to thank the whole of the Piatkus team for their help and support.

Preface

In this new book, which is revised from our earlier work *Sacred Healing*, we expand and develop the foundation material given in *Your Healing Power* and show you how to put the wisdom of the heart at the centre of your healing practice – to make it soul-based. This is the key to Spiritual Healing. (When Spiritual Healing appears in capitals throughout the book, it refers to the special method and teachings of the soul-based approach described herein).

Healing is evolving and we invite you to take part. First, let's look at what has been happening since the publication of *Sacred Healing* in 2001. It is very clear to us that the human family has been receiving a series of wake-up calls, in terms of the environment, climate change, the extinction of species, societal breakdown and alarming trends in human health. This last includes the statistic that one in three of us in the developed world suffers from some form of chronic disease. The situation certainly seems dire, but your interest in healing implies that you would like to play a creative role in addressing it. Dire situations usually announce a new phase in evolution, the driving force behind life.

It was a dire situation – chronic back trouble – which led Jack to spiritual healing. The treatment was so successful that he wanted to know how it worked! Since then we have spent much of the past 20 years researching, teaching and practising healing from our base in South Wales. Our work led us to join the National Federation of Spiritual Healers (NFSH) and we soon became national tutors, with Jack also working internationally. After writing two books on the subject, Jack's *Your Healing Power* was published in 1994 and has since become an international healing classic. Over the years we found that the root cause of the physical, emotional and mental symptoms of our clients was changing dramatically – a change which seemed to be reflected in national and global events. To find answers, we had to attune and listen to the voice of the client's soul.

THE VOICE OF THE SOUL

The whole point of human life is the manifestation of the soul *through* the personality, its body, mind and emotions. But what has been happening is that we now live according to the dictates of the personality alone. The voice of the soul is either not being heard or not being listened to. When disconnection from the soul occurs, we tend to live in a way which is actually not conducive either for human beings, all other life forms, or for the rest of the planet. This has led to a state of being we call 'soul malaise'. This is the effect on the individual.

Soul tries to draw our attention to this through our feelings, with the question: does this feel right? But when its voice is not heard it moves the question down through the levels of mind, emotions and the etheric to appear as stress, anxiety, mental ill health and emotional problems. Finally the question appears in the physical body as allergies and disease.

The second major effect of soul malaise is the effect on our planet. As part of cosmic evolution, Earth, like us, is evolving, but natural planetary changes are being aggravated by human interaction with the environment. Some people even feel that many disastrous planetary changes are the consequences of negative human thought and behaviour. Whatever their causes, we are increasingly experiencing the dramatic effects of the environmental and climatic transformations needed to restore natural balance.

Thus soul malaise is affecting the planet, the Earth Family (those other beings with whom we share the planet), as well as human individuals, families, societies and even countries. Healing is evolving because all these situations actually originate at a spiritual level. There is a need for alignment with the soul. The cure, then, cannot rest in pharmaceuticals and medical intervention alone – no matter how well intentioned. Soul malaise is healed by reunion with our spiritual reality, by reconnection with that Oneness which is the Source. That is what we hope this book will teach you to do.

HEALING SOUL MALAISE

The pain and distress we feel as we experience today's challenging situations are a call from the soul. It is addressed directly to our hearts. This awareness happens in the heart centre – that energetic centre of love which is the 'dwelling place' of the soul. Our focus must begin here – and not in our minds – if we are to respond to its summons.

The times we are living in demand a big leap forward in what healing now has to address, and in how to address it. The world needs healers who are aware of, and who can respond therapeutically to, the myriad symptoms of soul malaise. This new approach has to be soul-based. Just as the male or female shaman has always been central to the health and well-being of indigenous groups, so the evolving spiritual healer is now needed to play this crucial role in today's societies.

THE HEALING TRILOGY

Our response to this call of the soul is a trilogy of healing handbooks for the interested reader. We all have the power to take action and these three books describe how to do it. The first, entitled *Your Healing Power*, provides you with the basic foundation material for healing practice. It contains much of the NFSH course material Jack helped to devise, and is considered the best guide available on how to help and heal other people.

To emphasise that healing is evolving and to help you to respond to the call from the soul, we have reissued the second book, *Sacred Healing*, in the revised format of *The Spiritual Healing Handbook*. This has at its core the evolutionary nature of healing and how the soul cannot be excluded from the healing session. It provides the practical tools of Spiritual Healing and helps you to reunite with the Source, your higher power. It can be used as a guide to spiritual growth and self-healing, as well as deepening your work as a practitioner.

Jan's case studies of people she has worked with show how all other interventions can fail until the soul malaise of the patient is addressed. *The Spiritual Healing Handbook* actually presents a model for future living – how we live and how we relate to one another. It also raises issues about how soul has to be put back into education, business, government, social services and health care.

The soul-based approach of *The Spiritual Healing Handbook* encourages you to re-examine your attitudes and expectations – to your work, to those you work with and about outcomes. The approach emphasises the importance of your preparations, attunement and your own state of being. When the healing session is seen as a meeting of souls, who or what is a 'patient' or 'client', what is a 'cure' and what does 'healing' mean? Above all, what does it mean to be part of Oneness? As well as providing you with practical tools, *The Spiritual Healing Handbook* guides you to find your own answers to such questions.

Many cases of soul malaise can be treated by Spiritual Healing. However special forms of healing are now needed to reach out to the societal and environmental problems that are a fact of life in the 'global village'. Again, this aspect of the evolutionary nature of healing is addressed with Jack's important new third book of the trilogy, *The Distant Healing Handbook*. This complete manual teaches you how to send healing energy when the subject is at a distance from you – to individuals, animals, your pets, the environment and local and global issues – whether working by yourself or with a group.

Jack and Jan Angelo, July 2007

Introducing
Spiritual Healing

1

The Soul-based Approach

As we pointed out in the Preface, like all living systems, healing is evolving. Healing has had to evolve because people are becoming more spiritually aware and more aware of soul malaise. Friends, readers and contacts from around the world have been signalling to us that they are ready to work more deeply with the challenge presented by today's problems. So we invite you to further develop your healing channel and move to new levels of working.

From the Spiritual Healing perspective, 'spiritual' means everything to do with soul, or Higher Self, and the Source. The Source is what some call 'God'. Spirit is the energy of the Source. This is our reality – we are spiritual beings exploring what it means to be human. To live life consciously as a human being, we are multidimensional. In addition to our spiritual selves, we have mental and emotional aspects and a physical body to travel in the physical universe. But our spiritual reality means that we are able to align with the Source, to channel the healing energies that can operate at every level of our multidimensional being and to extend this ability to the rest of the Earth family and the environment.

Our experience working with groups and giving workshops, as well as in our one-to-one practices, has convinced us that growing numbers of people feel the need to bring the spirit and the Source into all aspects of their lives.

Whether you are an existing hands-on healer, a complementary therapist, a health professional, facilitator or trainer, *The Spiritual Healing Handbook* is designed and written for everyone who wants to further their spiritual development and healing abilities. We will show you how to create a soul-based healing session, starting with the basic essentials and moving on to the advanced techniques of the method. You will discover:

- How to create the soul-based approach, to heal in a spiritual, soul-based way.
- How to reconnect with the sacred aspect of yourself – your inner spiritual reality – or how to strengthen the link you already have.
- The various systems through which the soul operates. These are the subtle energy bodies which process the mental, emotional and etheric aspects of your life, as well as the energetic polarities of your physical body and skeleton. You will learn about the crucial role that the subtle energy centres (chakras) play in linking the systems to form the total human and in processing all aspects of your experience.
- How both healer and patient are further empowered within and outside the healing session in the meeting of souls.
- The role of Spiritual Healing in the rituals of birth and death, healing and loss.
- How Spiritual Healing can help bring the sacred and the wisdom of the soul into your community.

Part of being human is the fact that most of us can become so overwhelmed by physicality and physical life that we separate ourselves from spiritual reality and become convinced that we are simply our personality, with its body, mind and emotions. Separation may be so firmly established that we no longer see the spiritual in other people and we no longer see the natural world as the unveiled face of God. There are times when the sense of separation can become too hard to bear, leading to internal and external strife, manifesting as disease and unhappiness, intolerance and aggression.

At the beginning of this new millennium, the real healing of our disconnection must begin with causes rather than symptoms. These are soul-based, as our distant ancestors understood.

THE SPIRITUAL HEALING PERSPECTIVE:
SOME HISTORY

Until modern times, human life was tribal, in the setting of a specific natural environment – we were indigenous, social people. The healing activities of indigenous peoples around the planet today show that, since ancient times, techniques have been developed by individual men and women, according to their personal links with the spiritual or sacred. Very often healing is a communal activity, where ritual and ceremony are used to facilitate individual and group healing. One of the great authorities on myth, Joseph Campbell, considered that a primary function of ritual and ceremony was to give depth and form to human life, so that it should not be confined to religious activities alone. In his book *Coyote Medicine* (chapters 7 and 8), Dr Lewis Mehl-Madrona clearly describes how the ceremony of the sweat lodge is used in Native American medicine for both individual and group healing. 'People need ceremony,' he says, for 'ceremony creates the magic that allows healing to happen.' To illustrate these points, we include, in Chapter 18, the thrilling description of a Ju-hoansi healing ceremony.

Prominent amongst these indigenous activities is the laying on of hands, or healing touch. This tells us that hands-on healing is very ancient indeed. In some forms of shamanism, for example, healers were able to transmit power in this way after entering a trance state where healing power was said to have been the result of contact with the spirit world. Very often, in the same culture, healers demonstrated a strong bond with the spiritual, but here, the energy came directly from the Source. The people knew that not only was healing a sacred gift from this level of being, it was a sign that the Source was imminent and omnipresent. In recent times, the Native American healer and holy man, Frank Fools Crow, assured people that this indeed was the case. This last mentioned form of therapeutic activity is known in modern language as *spiritual healing*, where the energies of healing are believed to emanate from the Source.

Once our ancestors began to farm and to live in towns and cities, along with the development of writing (rather than oral tradition), healing and health care diverged into two main streams – indigenous or shamanistic forms and the techniques of the urban healer or physician. In the Western world, the ancient Greeks saw people as composed of spirit, mind and body and it was stressed that health could not be restored to the sick unless treatment addressed all these levels. This closely resembles the holistic or integrated approach which is becoming more accepted in the 21ˢᵗ century! But in the Greek and Roman world-view a profound split later developed where the gods were separate from humans, and humans were seen as separate from the natural world.

With the conversion of the Roman state to Christianity in the 2nd century CE, this world-view was enforced as a political, as well as a spiritual, reality. A person was still considered a being of spirit, mind and body, but the Church took over the care of the spirit leaving the care of the mind and body to the doctors – giving medicine the fractured view of a person from which it has not yet recovered. Western medicine still, to a greater extent, treats only the symptoms of the body – not of the mind.

Since indigenous forms of health care were linked to the sacred, these methods were seen as a threat to ecclesiastical power so that, by the middle of the medieval period (1100-1600 CE), hands-on healing outside of the Church was outlawed in the UK by a series of Witchcraft Acts. This attitude gradually spread throughout the world.

In the mid 17th century, the progressive disconnection of science from its ancient spiritual roots allowed the development of the mechanistic world-view, in which the human body was treated as a system of parts, each with basic mechanical functions.

But the darker sides of industrialization, and the birth of new economic philosophies, brought demands for freedom, especially in the realm of spirituality. Many Europeans fled to America where they felt they could live without the threat of persecution. By the middle of the 19th century people were demanding the freedom to practise hands-on healing.

To stay within the law, the new church of spiritualism was created. Spiritualists felt that they had recovered two important aspects of spirituality which had disappeared from Western culture – proof of life after death (through the work of clairvoyant mediums) and the natural ability to heal. In recent times, the work of the spiritualist churches, and the campaigning zeal of the great British healer, Harry Edwards (1893-1976), undoubtedly returned hands-on healing to the people. His mass healing demonstrations in venues such as the Albert Hall challenged the status quo, but the last Witchcraft Act was not repealed until 1951. In the US too, healing has been illegal unless practised within a 'church'.

In 1955 Edwards co-founded the National Federation of Spiritual Healers (NFSH), a non-denominational organization designed to represent healers, liaise with government and medical bodies and to present healing to the public. But it was not until a year after his death in 1976 that spiritual healing was recognised as a therapy by the British Medical Association. Today, the NFSH is the world's leading healing organization with an extensive training programme and a network of centres around the UK and abroad. The Harry Edwards Healing Sanctuary, founded by him in 1946, has recently become the new headquarters of the NFSH.

Spiritual healing is totally natural, but centuries of persecution and misrepresentation have left a legacy of confusion in the public mind – about healing, as well as the terms *spiritual* and *spirituality*. We want to emphasize that a person does not have to be a spiritualist or belong to any religion in order to develop and practise as a healer.

It is not surprising that, with the developments in complementary health care over the past thirty years, there has come a reconnection with, and a fresh understanding of, indigenous and shamanistic forms of healing, with their emphasis on the role of personal development and spirituality in human and planetary health. As the human spirit struggles to overcome the dehumanising aspects of modern life, we are realising that many indigenous peoples have been the guardians of a natural spirituality that is universal, timeless, and available to all of us today.

A MEETING OF SOULS

Our researches into the indigenous roots of spiritual healing led us to work with Native American medicine people in the UK. In 1996 we accepted an invitation to visit their country, and during a month of travelling the Southwest, we spent time with the Navajo and the Indians of the Pueblos. One afternoon we decided to visit Window Rock, a place sacred to the Diné (Navajo) people where they had set up their National Center in the 1930s. Signs along the road exhorted travellers to 'Drive in Beauty'. We pulled into the Center, only to find the place deserted. On one side of the sandy clearing, a pink sandstone ridge, weathered smooth over thousands of years, towered above a few juniper trees, forming the northern wall of what seemed like a natural cathedral. Erosion had created a huge round space in this wall, some 15 metres (about 45 feet) across, like a rose window through which the blue Arizona sky glowed.

As we sat on the pink earth, we both felt our hands buzzing and held them up to sense the energies. I found myself thinking: It's so peaceful here…like some kind of ancient healing temple. Jan smiled back at me, as if reading my thoughts. The afternoon sun blazed. The scent of juniper and sagebrush wafted by. In the silence, I was aware of a surge of energy within me. I realized, with a start, that it had begun with a feeling of being totally at one with the place, and then the place and I seemed to dissolve and disappear. But in that brief moment of transcendence I knew that it was an energy which could heal, in the widest and deepest sense.

A shadow interrupted the next thought. We looked up to see a smiling brown face. Michael introduced himself as a Navajo who had missed his chance to be a guide that afternoon. The bus full of European tourists had left without him. Could he spend some time with us and tell us some Navajo stories? We were delighted when he sat down with us.

He invited us to join him in a simple healing ceremony. 'You don't have to make a traditional sand painting, but you do need to prepare.' Michael caressed the ground with flattened palms, chanting in a high, gentle voice. 'The Earth loves to be sung to,' he smiled, drawing a square shape in the sand with a circle inside. Finally, he made a dot in the centre. 'Now we are ready.' He prayed aloud, 'Great Spirit, I call to you. We give you thanks for this opportunity ... I ask for a blessing on these souls. I ask for a healing for these people ...'

Time seemed to have stood still and yet the sun was beginning to lose its intensity when Michael looked straight into it, raised his arms and chanted in a high voice. 'Beauty before us, Beauty behind us, Beauty above us, Beauty below us, Beauty all around us. May we walk in Beauty!' He explained that, for the Diné, to 'walk in Beauty' was not simply being out in a beautiful landscape, it was a state of consciousness – the state of realizing the Source present in all things and in all people.

Driving back to New Mexico, we found ourselves talking about the healing ceremony – its simplicity, its directness, its prayerfulness, and how Michael had appeared so auspiciously. Jan looked ahead, as the headlights reached into the gathering dusk. The mountains were beginning to merge with the darkness of the desert. 'It was a meeting of souls,' she said. 'That's what healing is about.'

THE IMPACT ON OUR EVOLVING PRACTICE

During our time in the US we witnessed many other kinds of sacred ceremony and learned of doctors who were incorporating healing rituals into their regular practice. Their experience was that, by addressing the spiritual needs of patients, they had discovered a vital part of the healing process which had previously been missing.

When our connection with the Earth and with the spiritual/subtle realms is celebrated, the work place becomes a space where heaven and earth meet. Through conscious awareness of this, healer, patient and the sacred become one – and soul-based healing begins.

These meetings and our encounter with Michael in the desert had a profound impact on us. It highlighted the ways in which our healing practice had been evolving. Over the years, the emphasis had shifted from addressing the presenting physical, emotional or mental conditions of patients to their need for alignment with the soul.

Today, our practice has become a sacred ceremony where the souls of all concerned are invited to attend. The preparations for the ceremony imbue the healer and the healing space with a sacred consciousness. This offers the healer the opportunity to be guided at a soul level and to conduct the healing 'ceremony' from this level. It also invites the patient to be present in this way.

This has led to insights into the soul journey, the communication systems used by the soul, the place of the sacred in the use of therapeutic tools, the role of the sacred in giving meaning to life rituals and its potential for recreating community. The goal is to open up the person's consciousness to their deep and true nature so that this is liberated to express itself through the life of the individual. *The Spiritual Healing Handbook* offers you the opportunity to work with these discoveries.

THE SOUL-BASED CAUSES OF ILL HEALTH

During 20 years of practice, we have explored the causes of illness and suffering in patients and the distress and unhappiness in group members presented during training. Though there were often many different secondary causes, in every case there was a partial or total disconnection from the spiritual dimension of life. In spite of the fact that each person's unique reason for being human is soul-based, soul-designed and soul-directed, for so many, life has become soul-less.

If the expression of soul is inhibited, its energies cannot flow through the mind and body to empower and influence the life of the individual. The vital force which encourages and supports the life mission is missing. The individual is unable to exist in harmony with other people, the environment, and the Earth family. When such disconnection is the day to day experience of a person, it becomes a fundamental cause of ill health – for the individual, the community and the planet – it becomes soul malaise.

HEARING THE PATIENT'S STORY

In this way, some kind of distress or illness eventually initiates the meeting between healer and patient. Since the presenting conditions – whether mental, emotional or physical – are the different ways soul uses to communicate, it is important for the patient to become aware of and interact with what is being communicated.

This is done by encouraging our clients to tell their story, choosing whatever comes to mind. As the person talks, healing energy becomes focused on the content of the story – the presenting condition, life experience, relevant people and incidents, etc. As a result, the patient is able to enter the healing state free from mental and emotional turmoil. This creates a positive change in the patient's energy field.

In the telling of their story, the patient retraces their life journey, highlighting significant experiences and sharing reactions to them. The territory covered may be reviewed many times. Past journeying is also made visible. Gradually a life map begins to appear. The healer becomes a travelling companion, facilitating the healing needed for the effects of the journey to date and equipping the patient for the path ahead. Our book will teach you how to become such a healing companion, but, as we did, you may also find it helpful to acquire listening and awareness skills such as counselling.

SPIRITUAL HEALING AS THE WAY FORWARD

At the beginning of the new century, the emphasis in health care continues to be on addressing the symptoms of those conditions which the soul has created. Medical technology and pharmacology have created numerous means of relieving pain and suffering and of eliminating the symptoms of a condition as quickly as possible. These are valuable aids to recovery, but if the spiritual dimension is missing, the most important aspect of the patient is ignored.

When this is the case, the soul of the patient is never considered, consulted or listened to. Neither are the souls of those involved in the health care. No one is given the opportunity to become aware of or to understand the soul's purpose in the whole drama of life, ill health and death. This is why soul-based healing is so important – it gets to the very root of the problem.

Spiritual Healing offers a way forward to an integrated, soul-based model of health care for the future. We believe that working this way will lead to important discoveries about the art and science of healing, the healing environment and the causes of ill health. For you, the healer, it offers a therapeutic approach to making your healing more soul-based, which may also be a form of spiritual practice.

Healing at this level can be seen as a spiritual initiation in that it is an opportunity for the individual – healer or patient – to encounter the light of their own inner being. This is the force behind any transformation that might occur and is the important difference between the soul-based approach and any other therapy or form of medicine.

2

Working With This Book

GETTING STARTED

This book may be used by anyone who is looking for practical ways to bring the spiritual dimension into their life and work. If you are a healer or a complementary therapist, working with this book will enhance your experience and awareness, as well as providing a base line for more advanced practice. However, in conjunction with *Your Healing Power*, the material may also be used by those wishing to work with the Spiritual Healing model from the outset. If our chapter on Distant Healing resonates for you, *The Distant Healing Handbook* will introduce you to the full range of possibilities of working this way.

THE ACTION POINTS

The 53 Action Points we give you throughout this book guide you through the essential experience of Spiritual Healing, enabling you to work with the key themes and ideas presented in each chapter. They are the developmental tools which will broaden and deepen your awareness and understanding. Each has the dual function of enhancing practice as well as offering the opportunity for increasing spiritual and intuitive awareness.

You will find it very beneficial to have a basic knowledge of the subtle energy system and to have worked with the exercises in *Your Healing Power*. But for those new to the subject, when a particular concept is introduced, cross references will guide you to the more detailed information that follows in a later chapter. These concepts are also defined in the Glossary.

The text clearly specifies whether an Action Point is appropriate for the healer, the patient, someone interested in working with the principles, or a combination of these.

Take as much time as you need to properly absorb the effect of the material before moving on to a new topic. Make sure that you have given yourself enough space to complete each unit of practice. To avoid interrupting the flow of the work, in many cases you may find it helpful to make a recording of the instructions.

The way you attend to the practice and the experience of the Action Points will determine the quality of the process and outcome. Where an exercise asks you to visualise or 'see' something, this is simply using your natural ability to imagine. Never worry if you are unsuccessful at first in achieving a certain outcome in any of the Action Points. Keep up your practice and remain confident that the power of your intention, or the mental command, will ensure that it is taking place at some level of consciousness.

If you find you are tense or anxious during an exercise, stop. Follow a relaxation procedure and look after your breathing (refer to the breathing and relaxation exercises where necessary). Give yourself time to relocate consciousness in your still centre and start again.

Note: There are many people with disabilities who are healers. Wherever you find it necessary, please adapt the exercises to suit your situation.

Developing perception and looking after yourself

As you work with the book, you will find yourself becoming more sensitive and aware and the range of your perceptions will broaden. Learning to strengthen and trust your perceptions is reconnecting you with a level of awareness which was common to our ancient ancestors and which can enhance your life and your work. You should start to feel more confident and in harmony with others, the Earth and the Earth family. An attitude of open-heartedness and positive expectation will ensure your enjoyment of the material.

Increased awareness and sensitivity means that you must take care of yourself energetically. With this in mind, refer to the Action Points *Clearing the Energy Field, Closing Down* and *Protecting the Energy Field* in Chapter 4 so that you can use them straight away.

The Adventure of Self-Discovery

Self-discovery is the adventurous part of anyone's life journey. Experience confirms that development as a healer goes hand in hand with personal transformation. Absorbing the material and working with the Action Points will bring to the surface anything which needs healing, such as a past event. This is natural and should be seen as an indicator of progress, an opportunity rather than a problem. Love yourself enough to find a healer or a counsellor, to help you at this stage of your journey.

Where exercises may be carried out alone, to enhance inner development or to aid self healing, this is indicated in the text. But if you do decide to work alone, make sure that there is a trusted person, a healer or healing group with whom you can discuss your experiences. Ideally you should work with a partner or a group which is under the guidance of an experienced facilitator.

Confidentiality

In the exercises with a partner, confidentiality should be agreed within the context of your work together or within a group situation, whichever is appropriate. This honours what you have discovered about another person and what they have shared with you. When confidentiality is a stated boundary of the work, people feel safer and are more able and willing to share experiences.

SPIRITUAL HEALING AND TRAINING

A restoration of the sacred begins with the recognition of each other's spirituality so that training and practice acknowledge the spiritual dimension of the students, tutors and the work they will do together.

In some forms of spiritual healing the healer attunes to the Source and may or may not link with the soul of the patient. But the healer may then go on to depend on a learned technique alone and not be open to direction from the soul. In the soul-based approach of Spiritual Healing, the healer links with the Source *and* their own soul before engaging with any patients. Then, at the beginning of the healing meeting, the healer links with the soul of the patient. This is the 'meeting of souls' described earlier.

If you work in a caring profession, you are sensitive and aware. In our talks with many carers about their work and their working environment, they often describe a sense of something missing and a need to respond to the patient in some additional way. This may be an appropriate demonstration of love, such as compassion, but more often they refer to some kind of 'spiritual' response. Their training, however, may not encourage responses of this kind, nor reflect the need for an environment more conducive to healing. *The Spiritual Healing Handbook* validates such experiencing and outlines a sound framework for defining that 'something missing' while providing guidelines for safely incorporating it into whatever your practice may be.

While offering a challenging model to those who are providing training, the book also offers similar challenges to all other health care professionals to research what happens when this truly holistic, soul-based healing model is integrated into treatment, care, and attitudes to life, health, illness and death. If you are a trainer or facilitator, make sure that you are familiar with the material before using it with groups. Keep a note of what happens and how participants respond to the material.

Again, when confidentiality is a stated boundary of the work, people feel safer and are more able and willing to share experiences. With this in mind, if you are in a situation where a facilitator does not bring this up at the beginning of a piece of work, it is up to you to bring it to the attention of the facilitator and the group.

KEEP A JOURNAL

To make full use of the book, your own journal will be a useful record of what happens. You can add your comments, insights, dream material and anything else which seems to have a bearing on your progress. Sometimes your drawings, paintings or some other kind of creative work will be more expressive than words.

Looking back on your journal is a rewarding experience. You will have a fascinating personal record which shows how you engaged with the book and in what ways you have made progress. You may also discover new abilities and new possibilities. Following the guidelines of the book will greatly increase your ability to function as a healer, safely, effectively and with confidence. Having learned how to help yourself, you will have a better understanding of how you can be of service to others.

Let's begin work by looking at the principles of Spiritual Healing.

The Principles

3

The Soul Journey

Mary was seeking help for the anguish caused by three failed IVF treatments. The procedures had been extremely stressful and she was exhausted. It was important to teach her some simple relaxation skills that would help her to begin the process of recreating a positive relationship with her body, which she felt had let her down.

Early in the first healing session, Mary slipped into a state of deep relaxation. The basic scanning procedures revealed the extent of her exhaustion and emotional pain. Her energy centres had all been adversely affected by her experiences. The process of rebalancing them was begun. While working, I intuitively sensed that there would be a pregnancy and that it would be by natural means. This was not shared with the patient.

After the session Mary said she felt more positive about trying for another baby and she would explore the possibility of funding for further IVF treatment with her doctor!

Two months went by when an excited Mary rang to say she was pregnant without any IVF treatment. She continued to have healing over the next three months, then missed her usual session. Her husband rang with the sad news that she had lost the baby.

This was a test for me too. I had received a soul message that Mary would become pregnant and assumed that she would have a baby. I was reminded that the message had stated there would be a pregnancy and this had in fact happened.

Six months passed before Mary returned. She wanted to heal her body and continue the relaxation exercises that she had found so beneficial. Once more, she slipped into a deep, healing sleep while I carried out the basic scanning procedures. The same centres called for healing energy.

Then, towards the end of the healing, Mary's arms began to rise into the air until her hands were some 30cm above her belly. She remained asleep, while her arms and hands seemed poised in the position of someone heavily pregnant. Wave after wave of healing energy flowed through her, soothing and healing the physical body, eventually moving into the emotional and mental levels. Slowly, Mary lowered her arms back to the healing couch. Her face looked sublime as tears of joy coursed down her cheeks.

At the end of the healing, she returned to normal waking consciousness. She announced that she knew she would have her baby. A soul had chosen her to be the mother.

Quite soon after the session, Mary became pregnant by natural means and nine months later a perfectly healthy baby boy arrived to join the Earth family and begin his journey.

It was the right time on Mary's journey for her to experience pregnancy and motherhood.

From the time of birth, incarnating souls begin to develop a new sense of self as they become conscious of their own physical identity. The new self, or personality (ego), is a combination of this consciousness, what it inherits from parents and experience of life around it. As the growing baby becomes more and more immersed in life, it still has awareness of and contact with the subtle levels of being, but by about the age of three the little person is almost entirely ego-conscious. From then on life experience will have a bearing on whether or not the personality will make contact with the soul and when this will happen.

There have always been exceptions to this 'forgetting', as if those who do remember where we have come from are the living witnesses or evidence for the rest of us. The metaphysical poet Thomas Traherne, who died in 1674, was able to remember the time in his mother's womb. In *The Preparative* he describes this experience and then recalls his consciousness of pre-existence:

Before I knew these hands were mine
Or that my sinews did my Members join ...
I was within
A House I knew not, newly cloath'd with skin.
Then was my Soul my only All to me,
A living endless Eye
Scarce bounded with the sky
Whose Power and Act and Essence was to see;
I was an inward sphere of Light

ONENESS, DUALITY AND DIVINE DICHOTOMY

Earth exists as a unique destination for the journeying soul. Human experience grows and deepens through the dual aspects of physical life that are available on Earth. For example, we can discover more about love through knowing fear and all that lies between the polar opposites of love and fear. Similarly, we can discover more about light when there is its opposite, darkness, and all that lies between. Our understanding of truth is expanded through the experience of untruth, and so on. Our interaction with and reaction to these experiences and perceptions provides unlimited opportunities for the unfoldment of soul as we explore every aspect of separation and relationship.

All this is possible because of what is known as 'divine dichotomy'. This means that while everything appears to be separate from everything else, at the same instant everything is what the Australian Aborigines graphically call 'Oneness', another name for the Source.

Oneness is the truth of being, so we are holistically and energetically linked to one another, part of one another, at one with all of animal, plant and mineral life, at one with the planet, the stars and all beings in the universe. Because of divine dichotomy we can have a sense of separation, but we are actually one with all that is and all that is is one with us.

An implication of oneness is that if we harm another being we harm ourself. This is the true reason for gifting the world with healing – we take care of other beings because we are one with them, our nature is love. Healers have chosen, as part of *their* soul journey, to express this love through service.

RECALLING THE EXPERIENCE OF ONENESS

When receiving healing patients experience Oneness. This is familiar to them. They have also testified that they have caught glimpses of oneness or felt moments of a spiritual reality, very often in ordinary everyday situations. This has heightened their feelings of joy, bliss or happiness and, conversely, anguish, stress or sickness.

Such experiences suggest that some kind of parting has taken place. This is the great separation from soul and the Source, which for many manifests as life devoid of the sacred. Patients' statements are soul telling us how it is. We validate them and encourage patients to do the same.

On reflection, most people can recall one or more transcendental or 'oneness' experiences, especially from the time of childhood. Here is one example:

When Jack was eight years old he was living in a convent. One Sunday the nuns took the children to a nearby forest for their usual afternoon walk. As they went along in pairs, Jack and his friend waited for a chance to escape from the party. When the nuns were looking the other way, the boys darted from the path into the trees and were soon out of sight.

They found themselves in the dark depths of the trees when Jack felt that something was about to happen. Ahead of them they could see the light of a clearing. Then, just as they were about to enter the clearing, Jack held his friend back. The red-brown form of an adult fox had slipped silently into the pool of sunlight before them. The fox looked straight ahead, sniffing the air, its bushy tail in line with its back.

Jack was happy and at peace in the shimmering presence of the fox. Then he felt absorbed by what was happening, as if he and the fox, the sunlight and the trees were suddenly one being and had become one light.

It seemed much later when his friend was tugging at his sleeve. 'It's gone. We'd better catch up!'

Jack was always grateful to his friend for not breaking the magical silence of that moment until the fox had disappeared.

Oneness is what we are, so when we do reconnect with this level of reality it may seem strangely familiar, like a distant memory. We know it. It has meaning for us. Oneness experiences have certain characteristics – time may seem to stand still and there may be a new awareness of light. There may be a feeling that everything is a part of us, giving a fresh sense of life and feelings of profound joy. These feelings permeate our whole being and are vividly remembered.

We have all had experiences like these. It is simply a matter of recalling them to recognize them again and to restore this as a core practice. The concept of Oneness and the experiencing of Oneness are central to Spiritual Healing. So the first exercise in the book takes you to a moment of sacred recollection.

ACTION POINT I Recalling an Experience of Oneness

Developmental tool – acts as a reference point during healing.

The experience of oneness confirms the presence of soul. This exercise may be used as a self-healing technique, promoting a sense of oneness, wholeness and belonging.

- Allow yourself to relax somewhere comfortable where you will not be disturbed. Take a few deep breaths into the belly, then let yourself breathe normally.

- You want to recall a moment when you felt totally present to yourself and at one with all things, or totally in the stillness of the moment, as was described earlier on in the example of Jack. Something may pop into your mind straight away. If not, allow yourself to drift back through time.

- Once an experience shows itself on your mental screen, just allow it to run through like a video.

- At the end of the exercise, give yourself a few minutes to rest in your recollections.

- Now make a note of the experience in your journal, or make a picture or some other creation that the experience inspires.

- Thank your soul for bringing the moment to your attention.

UNDERSTANDING SOUL COMMUNICATION AND LIFE PRESSURES

Your recollection of Oneness will carry you through the work ahead and continue to enrich your practice. Nevertheless, as long as oneness is just an idea rather than an experience, our identification with the personality alone can distance us from our reason for being here. But, as each person's life demonstrates, soul finds ways of awakening us to the truth of who we are.

The first clues appear in childhood. Think back to what first gave you joy, what made you giggle. Think back to what seemed vibrant, full of life and passion. Think back to an activity or a situation when you felt like this. This is soul telling us about ourselves. If we have found ways in life to resonate with these childhood feelings, we are probably on the right track, in tune with our soul mission. But if our current life seems to have none of these resonances, we are probably out of tune.

Through the medium of feelings, soul tells us that when things do not feel good it could be a signal that something needs to change.

Deep down, we know when we are in tune with soul. We say we know something in our 'heart of hearts'. This is where soul resides, in the heart centre of the subtle energy (etheric) body. But we can disregard the clues so that soul has to find another way to get through to us. It exerts pressure to expose us to spiritual realities, especially during adolescence. We are looking then for what is good and true, noble and passionate, soul qualities that we took for granted when we were small children. We may have been shocked if these qualities, or people representing them, were snatched out of our lives. In adolescence we have a chance to reclaim them.

As we grow older, if we do not remember our true self, soul exerts pressure on where we are most vulnerable. At a mental level it creates thoughts, images and dreams, and eventually mental distress. This may lead to mental breakdown.

At an emotional level, soul exerts pressure in the form of feelings, images linked to feelings, dreams linked to feelings and eventually emotional distress. This may lead to emotional breakdown. But breaking down is breaking through, tearing aside the veil, seeing through the illusion of separateness.

All the while, soul is making contact and trying to get us to reclaim our relationship so that we can experience and create who we really are. Finally, pressure may be exerted on the body so that various conditions of physical distress and ill health begin to manifest. Soul may even create a condition where we are literally stopped in our tracks on the journey and forced to take stock of our life.

HEALING AS INITIATION

Just as soul speaks to us through feelings, it also speaks through the language of the presenting condition. In Spiritual Healing the condition, whether spiritual, mental, emotional or physical, is not seen as a problem or something to get rid of.

Rather it is understood as a communication from soul, which only the patient can truly understand and interpret. The skills of the healer and the level of energy channelled are the tools used to help the patient to decode the message. As we explained earlier, the meeting between patient and healer is a meeting of souls. Two souls on their individual life journeys meet and, for a time, may journey together. It is a sacred meeting because it puts the patient and the healer in touch with their own souls. For the patient it may also be a meeting with the Source. This is the conscious or unconscious initiation of the patient, an introduction to the light within, where deep healing begins.

Thus the energetic exchanges that result from the healing session have repercussions on all levels of the patient's being. These repercussions determine how the healing takes place and what will be the outcome. Healing, which is a restoration of harmony, always takes place at some level, but that may not be in the form we have assumed it ought. The deepest healing occurs when the link with soul is so made that its power is released into the life of the patient, bringing profound changes for the good.

OUR SACRED RELATIONSHIP WITH EARTH

Some of these changes may be in our relationship with Earth. For we are not just journeying with other people; we also make the journey with the one who has provided the material for our physical bodies and a perfectly balanced natural setting in which we can explore and create who we are.

We have become part of the planet's evolution and part of the evolution of the animal, plant and mineral kingdoms. So, knowingly or unknowingly, we have developed a sacred relationship with the planet and the whole of the Earth family.

But today, the condition of Earth, the contamination of food and drinking water, signals a breakdown in this relationship. This mirrors the condition of human minds, emotions and physical bodies. The reflection in the mirror tells us that this is what happens when we lose our sense of the sacred and our unity with all things. The most graphic examples of this loss are sickness, the break-up of family life, the break-up of community, and breakdown in society.

But are we listening? Have we reached a stage on our journey when we are prepared to heed the call to stop and listen?

LISTENING TO THE LANGUAGE OF THE PLANET

Some people have understood that these signs are telling us that we have reached the point on Earth's journey, and on our own journey, where it is now a matter of urgency that we become more aware of our actions and take responsibility for their consequences. Just as our body signals to us – it is time to pay attention, this condition is telling you something important – Earth is signalling to us to wake up and realize that we have to take care of things and heal the sacred relationship.

To do this, we will need to be available to listen in a sacred manner. We need to listen more carefully for the guidance of soul and to act accordingly. We are not used to doing this. We are not used to listening to one another, and even less are we prepared to listen to the voices of the animals and birds, plants and trees, the rocks and the very place on which we stand. We have forgotten that spirit, the energy of the Divine, takes on many forms, that soul speaks through all forms and on all occasions.

There are too many diversions in modern life that prevent us from hearing these voices. We seem to have given our ears other things to hear and our awareness other things to attend to. So it will take some practice to listen in this new way. You can make a start with the following exercise:

ACTION POINT 2 Linking with the Earth

Developmental tool – encouraging awareness of and sensitivity to Earth energies.

This may also be used as a self-healing exercise that honours the role of Mother Earth in the healing of the physical body. Take some time out of your routine to pay your respects to Mother Earth.

- Out of doors, find a piece of ground where you can be for a while without being disturbed. This could be a garden, an area in your neighbourhood or you may feel called to a location elsewhere. Introduce yourself to the place. Take a good look at it.

- Take off your shoes and socks and walk on the ground with bare feet. If this is not possible, touch the ground with another part of the body. Thank the Earth for this feeling. Consciously breathe in the scent of the ground. Notice where the Earth meets the sky.

- Choose a place to lie down. Let your body relax into the ground and feel it supporting you. Give thanks to the Earth for her support.

- Think of how your body is made from the Earth and how Earth supplies the food to nourish and maintain your body. Give thanks for your Earth body and your Earth food.

- Allow yourself to be at peace with the Earth. Be open and aware. Allow the Earth to speak to you in some way.

- Another time, ask Earth what you can do to take care of her.

- Sit up and become aware of your feet and, when you feel ready, stand up and walk about slowly and gently with bare feet. Be aware of the ground under your feet. See if you notice anything that you may have missed at the beginning.

- Give thanks for this time with Earth and with this place before you leave.

- Later, see if there is anything you would like to put in your journal to mark the exercise.

We are one with Earth. Her life is our life. The state of the land reflects the physical state of the human. Every time that we work with the Earth in a sacred manner we do something to bring harmony to the human body and wholesomeness to the land.

SICKNESS HELPS US TO REMEMBER THE SACRED

In former times, people lived in harmony with the environment. They created rituals and ceremonies to celebrate and honour the relationship, to remind the people of their roots in the Earth. Thanks to the efforts of indigenous peoples to preserve natural spirituality and to share its wisdom, we are learning how to reclaim this important aspect of the sacred.

Because we may no longer have meaningful ways to remind us of the sacredness of being, we have evolved a way of drawing attention to this through ill health. Sickness may force us to give up a stressful lifestyle, to review the nature of our food and how it is produced, to look again at where and how we are living and working or to take responsibility for our individual effects on the environment.

Two fundamental causes of ill health

In the correlation between sickness and reclaiming the sacred, there are two fundamental causes of ill health or distress that might lead to ill health. The cases below are typical illustrations of how healing was able to help the patient to recognize these causes as a breakdown in their inner relationships. The first demonstrates the breakdown of a person's relationship with soul and the Source:

Audrey could not understand the overwhelming sense of grief that dominated her life. At 40 and a successful businesswoman, she seemed to have everything – a happy marriage, two great children, a dream home and financial security. She wanted for nothing. But she still felt that something was missing.

On the recommendation of a friend, Audrey decided to try healing. Perhaps healing would explain her sense of grief and what was missing. She described a recurring need to take up a new hobby, to learn a new skill or to join a new class. It had become something of a joke in the family, but Audrey needed to keep her mind active and her life full.

In her first session Audrey broke down as she experienced the energies of healing. The healing power of love achieved the much-needed reconnection with the sacred aspect of Audrey – her soul. This was what was missing. Her mind had driven her to keep busy with new 'projects' as a way of compensating for the missing sacred connection. Audrey's life reflected both her material security and her spiritual insecurity. It was time to make amends.

Healing continued to support Audrey as she explored ways of honouring and celebrating her sacredness.

The second case illustrates the breakdown of a person's relationship with Earth and the Earth family:

Simon always felt alone. He had learned to hide the pain of this so that neither his partner nor any of his friends knew of his deep distress. One day he had had enough and decided to seek help. Through tears he told how years ago his family had dismissed his cries for help. 'You'll grow out of it' and 'It's something everybody goes through' were typical comments he had received.

But, at 28, Simon had not 'grown out of it' and, if anything, the pain and sense of disconnection was now more acute. His health was undermined by the constant struggle to deny his pain and, no matter how successful he was in life, it was always there, like a reminder. What was this reminder about?

As part of his preparation to receive healing, Simon was invited to visualize his connection to Mother Earth via his feet. He was encouraged to relax and allow the ground to support him. More tears flowed as he described the feeling of the Earth rising gently beneath his feet. He felt as if he had been 'given permission' to enjoy this connection and, in doing so, he had received an overwhelming sense of comfort and relief.

'I heard a voice just like mine, speaking to me ... it said, "Realize this is your unique connection with Mother Earth and all beings. Enjoy this sense of connection. This is the truth of your connection with Oneness. Know that you belong."

Simon continued attending for healing to release the pain of years of disconnection from the sacred. Gradually, his life reflected his sense of reconnection. Whenever he felt alone he would consciously feel the Earth beneath his feet and remember his 'unique connection'.

The frequency and universality of such cases, coupled with the worsening state of the planet, indicates that the overall crisis for us, the Earth and the Earth family, is a spiritual one. Sickness is becoming transformative and that is why healing can no longer be just about addressing symptoms. This means that nothing less than a spiritual approach will properly address what needs to be healed. Spiritual Healing shows that, by accessing soul to provide wisdom and loving guidance, a new way forward can be found that will return us to a sacred way of being.

THE KEY CONCEPTS

As we saw in Mary's story, life begins with the arrival of soul. Birth signals a new stage of the journey. During one's lifetime the impulse of soul will be experienced many times. Soul energies are released, prompting endings and signalling new beginnings. We will experience many 'births' created by soul impulse during our journey. This manifests as the need to make changes in relationships, lifestyle, career choices and geographical location. Spiritual Healing is a way of honouring and charting this process, and of facilitating the continual response to the call of soul.

To ensure that they can work with the two fundamental causes of ill health, healers practising Spiritual Healing embody the following key concepts:

- the therapeutic approach is soul-based and soul-centred
- the approach affirms the spiritual nature of all beings
- we are spirit (as soul) inhabiting a physical form
- we are energy beings
- we are on our unique journey of experience, learning and expression
- ill health and well-being are integral parts of the soul journey and can be identified as the communications of the soul
- healing the self is healing the whole
- healing and service to others is the natural outcome of understanding oneness.

This way of working arises from the needs and pressures of the new century. The Piscean Age appealed to the individual to develop the heart, to open to love and to find ways of expressing that love for the benefit of all. The Aquarian Age offers a deeper expression of that love to those who journey now. As we honour who we truly are and continue to align ourselves and our life ways with our sacred identity, we collectively draw this spiritual vision to Earth.

Ponder how we have chosen to be present on the Earth at this time of a major shift in consciousness, that we have chosen to be of service to the Earth and her peoples – to participate in grounding the spiritual vision for humanity. This is the call. This is the invitation. Spiritual Healing is a contribution to the grounding of the vision.

4

The New Healer

On the night of 27 November 1989, a blizzard raged over the Pine Ridge Indian Reservation. In his little cabin, the great Lakota healer and holy man, Fools Crow, passed over, having lived for 99 years.

A week later, at the time of his burial service, the skies cleared and over 500 mourners followed the brown-and-white spotted horse, which carried his warbonnet on a star quilt edged with red.

A nephew of Black Elk, Fools Crow was Ceremonial Chief of the Teton Sioux and a true leader of his people. His whole life of healing and service was a rich example and a great source of power that continues to radiate into the world today.

Frank Fools Crow said that anyone who was willing to live the life he led could do the things he did. This was a life devoted to Great Spirit (the Source), the (spirit) Helpers, and the people. He demonstrated the spiritual truth that great healing ability is the natural outcome of such a life of devotion.

Fools Crow used to describe a person's healing channel as a 'hollow bone'. The life ways of the healer were designed to create this hollow bone and to keep it as clear and uncluttered as possible.

Fools Crow's roots were deep in the Lakota tradition of sacred living.

Many feel that his passing marked the end of a way of life whose spiritual power produced so many healer warriors and holy people of both sexes. But, since 1989, the story and example of that great healer has lit a fire in the hearts of many young Lakota and people outside the US.

Interest in indigenous spirituality continues to grow and we are witnessing a new relationship with other spiritual groups and forms of spirituality from around the world, including shamanism, exploration of the goddess, natural spirituality, creation spirituality, and so on. These relationships and explorations are part of a movement to recover and reclaim a sacred way of life through a more enlightened contact with and understanding of indigenous sacred ways.

THE INDIGENOUS HEALER

Indigenous healers come from the community where they live. They are born with healing ability close to the surface and they enjoy a close relationship with the natural world. These characteristics are soon noticed and steps are taken within the community to foster and develop the young medicine people, who may be male or female.

They are encouraged to develop their own link with the Source, their own vision and their own spiritual power as a healer and as a person through their communion with nature, prayer, meditation and ceremonial practice. Healing procedures and knowledge are learned by being in touch with and being taught by their inner teacher and the Source. By means of this soul-guided way, they discover that the Source has infinite means of expression and communication through the planet, the animals and plants, the spirit world and, most of all, through themselves and their own abilities. The developing healer nurtures an affinity with certain of the Source's helpers (which may be spirit teachers and guides and power animals) and, through the bond of unconditional love, these lines of communication make special patterns of energy available to each healer's field of work. Through these links, the healer is drawn to areas of practice that feel natural, comfortable and stimulating.

Time has shown that this individual way of revealing the healer within is natural and effective. But it is important that experienced healers and other spiritual people of the community are always on hand to nurture, support and guide where necessary. This is the way the healers of Andean Peru, for example, are encouraged to develop.

The indigenous healer learns to trust the voice of soul, their intuition and inner vision, and their developing awareness enables them to confirm the appropriateness of intuitive guidance. In the indigenous context, the healer is a sacred person who brings about harmony wherever it is needed – in conditions of ill health, in people, in plants and animals, in planetary locations and situations.

Indigenous peoples believe that the global network of spiritually-centred people is preserving the world, acting as an energetic bulwark against the depradations of industry, commerce and technology that currently threaten all forms of life. The healer is therefore honoured as a person who is a gift to the community, the planet and the whole Earth family.

Indigenous Principles And The New Healer

Many of the indigenous aspects described earlier are characteristics that we encourage in the development of the New Healer. For example, the indigenous principle that everyone has the potential to access their own unique inner guidance has great relevance for anyone looking to develop as a person or as a healer. Whatever stage you feel you may be at in your work as a healer or on your journey as a seeker, consider whether any indigenous ways resonate for you. Perhaps you could try some of them yourself. They may be offering you new challenges. They may be asking you whether you go within for guidance or rely on your knowledge and experience alone.

Whether born into an urban forest or an urban desert, the new healers have come to serve all the people, the Earth, and the Earth family. Their agenda is nothing less than a realignment of the human with the sacred in all areas of life – a return to Oneness.

New Healer Qualities And Being Creative

The healer is heart-centred, listening to the voice of soul, rather than centred on the solar plexus, listening to the voice of mind. In terms of health care, the focus is less on human degeneration and more on each person's journey of transformation; less on fear and more on love.

By returning to soul-guidance and to Oneness, the healer develops a healing state of consciousness where their energy field itself becomes a healing presence. No one can be in a healing presence like this without something constructive happening. The New Healer knows that patients have their own inner reason for their condition and their own answer. Further, that soul selects those energies that will be most effective for that particular condition on that particular occasion. The healer's role is to create an environment where the healing presence can manifest, and to co-operate with and facilitate the energetic process. This is the creative role of the New Healer.

A need to fix the condition is uncreative and would mean that the healer never lives in the now because now needs to be changed. Consciousness is projected to then, in the past or future, where things are better. In the uncreative mode, patients and healers cannot accept things as they are. The focus is on what the patient should become.

Thus, anxieties about what should be done or put right interfere with creativity, our awareness of what we are doing and our ability to tune into what needs to be done. Once the flow of healing begins, if we remain fixed on an idea such as making the patient feel better, we lose contact with the healing opportunities that soul reveals. We interfere with the energetic flow and set about manipulating energy. This is the antithesis of the soul-based approach.

Moving with the rhythm of healing affirms a soul-state that exists independently of the individual. This rhythm of the soul is the force with which the creative healer co-operates and interacts. In this way, the creative healer becomes a means for the expression of soul.

The healer holds this view and builds the healing relationship upon it, supporting the difficulties the patient's personality may have in accepting rhythm of the soul – the healing function of the condition.

THE HEALING FUNCTION OF THE CONDITION

In the soul-based approach of Sacred Healing, the healer is journeying with the patient, bearing witness to the patient's experience of life throughout the healing process. The healer works with the presenting condition, acknowledging that it is soul's best way of describing the present within the context of the soul journey.

The healer understands that every condition or problem that a patient brings is what they have chosen as their way towards integration with their real self. Even confusion is welcomed as a situation in which the patient is seeking an understanding of the self.

A crisis is an opportunity to work and grow with the will of soul, or the Source, and the person who asks for help extends this opportunity to the healer. In this way the healer comes to recognize and welcome the creative function of the presenting condition, and accepts the invitation to partner the individual at this point of the journey.

The healer is present for the patient, without judgement or expectation. The healer is not there to take something away before the patient has had the chance to gain insight into the condition. The healer is the therapist, in the true sense of the word, who waits upon the God within, providing that therapeutic place of light where soul can come through and take the leading role in the patient's life (from the Greek *therapeuein*, to minister to).

LISTENING TO THE SACRED LANGUAGE OF HEALING

According to the codes of conduct drawn up by various healing bodies, such as the Confederation of Healing Organizations (CHO), the British Complementary Medicine Association (BCMA) and the National Federation of Spiritual Healers (NFSH), the healer should not make a medical diagnosis. Quite rightly, it should be left in the hands of doctors. However, a more fundamental reason for avoiding medical diagnosis is that the healer is there to listen to soul as it speaks, to honour the patient's experience of the condition, not to create limitations by naming it.

This allows the healer to bear witness to the thousand-and-one ways that soul finds to speak to us through the presenting experience. We do not fear the experience so we do not need to have power over it. We do not need to contain it so we do not need to confine it to the name of a condition.

The New Healer has to learn how to think with the heart rather than the head so that head comes to mean *focus* rather than thinking. They learn how to listen to the patient, remaining alert to the meaning behind every experience.

As the patient tells their story in their own way, some medical history may well be revealed. What is important, from the healing point of view, is that which the patient wants to reveal, how, when and in what order it is revealed. For the patient is talking about their relationship with the condition, the relationship with themselves, their life journey and with soul.

In this listening mode, the healer discovers what is important to patients. The healer is there as a mirror to allow them to see what is important to them – in effect, to see themselves, and to support them in their process of understanding their life and in re-establishing their link with the sacred.

While being alert and aware, the healer is also totally relaxed. In this way the healer is being present to both soul and the patient as a person. Alertness is needed to avoid moving out of the healing consciousness prematurely. This can happen when the healer asks, for example, 'What is your problem?', which carries the message, 'I am separate from you because you are the one with the problem'. Similarly, anxiety about the state of the patient can cause the healer to move out of healing consciousness.

Every patient has a unique story, which tells of adventures, triumphs and disasters, and reactions to life. On each occasion, the way the story is told reflects how the patient is experiencing their journey at that moment. When patients describe their experience, they are indicating where they seem to be at that point in time.

When they say, 'I think ...', they are talking about their thoughts and the state of their mind. When they say, 'I feel ...', they are talking about their feelings and their emotional state.

These phrases are the sacred language of healing to which healers need to be alert because this is soul's way of presenting the situation. The emphasis or frequency of the phrases gives a sense of weighting to the patient's perception of what is happening. Here is a way of looking at this:

ACTION POINT 3 The Sacred Language of the Soul – Weighting

Developmental tool – promoting the ability to listen in a sacred manner.

This exercise may also be used as a tool for self-healing to encourage a sacred dialogue about life experience.

- You will need a partner. Sit with each other as in a healing consultation. Your partner is the 'patient'. Prepare yourselves to be wholly aware by checking your posture. It should be comfortable with the feet flat on the floor, and the arms and legs uncrossed. Take several breaths to help relax the body and bring focus. See yourselves surrounded by the light of protection.

- The 'patient' talks about a current life challenge. You, the 'healer', listen with your whole being. Where and how are you experiencing your partner's words and your partner's presence?

- Try to experience the sacred language of the patient. Is your partner emphasizing feelings, thoughts or expressing the impact of the condition on the body or life itself?

- What is the patient's relationship to this challenge? Do you detect an issue of love and/or power, or lovelessness and/or powerlessness?

- After five minutes, thank your partner and offer what has been experienced by you.

- Swap roles and repeat the exercise.

- Compare notes. What do you now think 'weighting' means? How might weighting represent the location of the life challenge or condition within a level of physical, emotional or mental experience?

Weighting is about recognizing where, energetically, patients need help in processing their experience. The healer's job is to help patients 'unhook' from where they are weighted. This is what the healing will begin to do. During the healing session, all the information about weighting can be compared with the sensing and healing scans to see if they match up energetically.

By listening to the sacred language of healing, the healer becomes aware that every patient is a physical being, an etheric being, an emotional being, a mental being, and a spiritual being, and that each of these levels of the person has something to contribute to the story of their lives. (The functional relationship of these aspects of being is described in Chapter 9, Sacred Mind – Sacred Feeling.) The sacred language of healing is more than the patient's words, it is the entire communication during the whole of the healing process, of which the session is a part.

Awareness Of The Subtle Energetic State

Attunement information, such as that obtained in Action Point 3, coupled with the information from the healing procedures (see Chapter 14, The Sacred Meeting), provides an energetic picture of the patient at the time of the healing session. This energy picture does not have a name, but is nevertheless a diagnostic aspect of the healing process. This is quite different to a medical diagnosis where, after assessing symptoms, a condition is named, and pharmaceutical and technological help is directed according to the current level of medical knowledge about the named condition.

Spiritual Healing is a form of subtle energy medicine in which energetic diagnosis is not an informed guess about a probable medical condition, but an awareness of the subtle energetic state of the patient and openness to the direction of soul in bringing about harmony within the subtle energy system. (Detailed information on this system follows in Chapter 7, The Light Body.)

Holding The Patient In The Light

The healer is only able to act as a transmitter of the light (the healing energies), because they can be in that state of consciousness. The healing state is a consciousness of Oneness, which is the same as being soul-centred. In looking at the total energetic picture of the patient, the quality of the energy may be perceived as the quality of light within the energy field. Patients' statements about their condition, whether about a pain, a sensation or a state, are statements about their reaction to the absence of light, the diminishing or curtailment of the light or a change in the quality of light within their field.

Once the patient is engaged in the healing process, whether physically present or at a distance, the healer must be able to hold them energetically on all levels so that the light can be brought to bear at the level or levels to which it is needed.

The great mystic and pioneer in the study of energy medicine, Alice Bailey, considered that human sickness was 'the absence of light'. In our experience, until the right quality and quantity of light (as healing energy) has been brought to bear on the presenting condition, there is no true healing. This is why the healing encounter with the Source is often referred to as 'enlightenment'.

THE NEW HEALER'S ROLE

The New Healer finds ways to open and develop links with the Source, their own soul and the spirit world. By doing this, intuition and the healing channel – the 'hollow bone' – are developed so that teaching, guidance and assistance are received in the same way as they are received by indigenous healers. When this knowledge and experience is applied with love, they become the wisdom base of healing practice.

Every healing encounter provides an opportunity to glimpse the truth of who we really are. As we have explained, healing is ultimately an initiatory experience, though this should be seen in the context of a therapeutic approach. If healers see their practice as a therapy, they should regard it as a complementary therapy and must be prepared to work alongside all other forms of health care, especially conventional medicine, according to a code of conduct such as those drawn up by the CHO and the NFSH (1999). We consider that the healer's role is, above all, to facilitate the meeting of souls.

The New Healer is not interested in making spiritual healing exclusive or in an elitist hierarchy of caring. Instead they are forging relationships with orthodox medicine and other health care professionals who are dedicated to the creation of an integrated model of health care, with the patient's spiritual reality at its heart. The New Healer practises Oneness.

We have set out above how the principles of Spiritual Healing are embodied in the New Healer. These determine what healers will need to be able to do to carry out the demands of their role. Later in the book we discuss how the work of the New Healer will help to create the basis of sacred community.

Being a healer is a calling that has to be worked at, cherished, developed and celebrated with passionate energy. Moreover, the quality of the light and love we offer another person will not simply depend on the training we have had or the hours we have put in, but rather is the outcome of who we are, how we honour our own life journey and who we are in the process of creating. For the New Healer, like the indigenous healer, this means being in special relationship with soul and the Source.

In Chapter 5 we go on to show how the New Healer can create this special relationship and create a sacred way of being that inspires practice.

5

A Way of Being

Restoring the sacred brings healing and makes healers of us. This chapter is about how to restore the sacred in your own life so that you can work with the principles and objectives of Spiritual Healing. We shall look at how to develop healing consciousness through the creation of a healing way of being. The core practice is to be centred, in communion with your own sense of Oneness (remember Action Point 1, which gave you a recollection of this). This creates and defines the healing channel, and has a direct bearing on how you approach and carry out the work.

THE SACRED ELEMENTS OF THE BODY

The Action Points in this chapter are ways of bringing you to your own sense of Oneness and remembrance of this. Let's start with the body and its sacred elements.

Relating to water

Most of our body is made of water so we have a close relationship with this life element. We can make this relationship more conscious by recalling how vital it is to life. Symbolically, it represents the emotions and, especially in dreams and visions, can guide us to an understanding of our emotional state.

Water is not only the best medium for cleansing the physical body – its therapeutic properties are also well known. This is because water is a superb carrier of subtle energies (those energies that vibrate faster than the speed of physical light, including healing energies), especially the life force. Since the earliest days of our history, water has been used in a sacred manner.

ACTION POINT 4 The Healing Power of Water

The Action Points in this chapter encourage us to celebrate life as a spiritual being and to develop sensitivity to the interrelatedness of all things. They may also be used as self-healing activities, promoting a sense of oneness, wholeness, health and well-being.

- Fill a bowl with water or go to a safe source of water such as a clear shallow pool or stream. If water is needed as a cleanser or to clear away worry, anxiety or stress, see it filled with silver light. As you splash it over you, realize that the silver energy does the work of cleansing or clearing your body and emotional energy field. Thank water for its help.

- If you feel the need of a tonic or refresher, explain your need to the water. See the water filled with a brilliant light. Notice what you sense the colour to be. Your intention will allow the subtle energy to blend with the energy of the water. Splash it over you, especially over the face and neck. Thank water for its help.

After washing in the morning, sip a little fresh water. Thank it and bless it as you recall its need for purity and freedom.

We are one with water. Its life is our life. The state of water on the planet reflects the emotional state of the human. Every time we work with water in a sacred manner we do something to bring harmony to human emotions and to return purity to water.

Relating to the sun and air

Once ablutions are complete, before eating, it is time to greet the day. Try to do this outdoors if possible. But even if the weather does not allow this, the new day is still there to be greeted and its sacred promise acknowledged.

The sun represents the cosmic sun, the light and warmth of the Source. The next exercise allows you to interact with the sun, the element of fire and with the element of air.

ACTION POINT 5 The Seven Breaths of Greeting

Developmental tool – promoting sensitivity to the cycles of giving and receiving.

- Face the direction of the dawn, the place of the rising sun, standing or sitting, and relax the body, using the breath to help the process of relaxation. Feel your body fully connected to the Earth.

- Give thanks for the previous night, whatever kind of night you have had. Be aware that the source of energy and the promise of each day is within you.

- Whether you can see the sun or not, its rays are beaming towards you. Allow them to bathe your body in light. Give thanks to the sun for its nourishing energies. Give thanks for the new day. You, the sun and the new day are one.

- Feel the air around you. Become aware of your breath and the fresh air entering your nostrils and filling your lungs. Notice how your whole body takes joy in the breath of the day.

- Now, as you breathe slowly and normally, raise your arms, with the hands palms up as if the rays of the sun can bathe them.

- In your position of thanks and greeting, take seven deep breaths down into the belly. As you exhale, visualize the life force in the air moving powerfully into the various parts of your body and energy field in the following sequence:

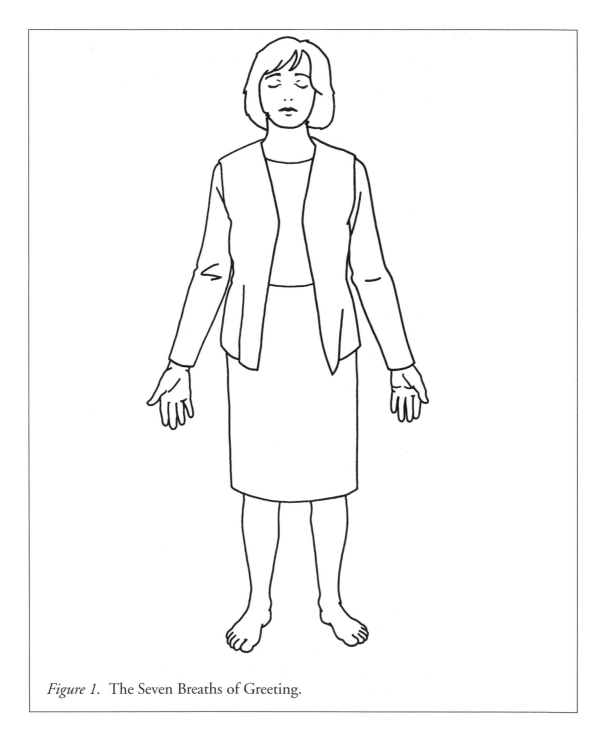

Figure 1. The Seven Breaths of Greeting.

- On the first breath, as you exhale, visualize the life force in the air moving down the length of your spine, filling it with life and relaxing the muscles of your back.

- With the second breath, as you exhale, take the life force down into your pelvis and legs, allowing it to relax the muscles of these parts.

- With the third breath, as you exhale, take the life force into the shoulders and arms, allowing it to relax the muscles.

- With the fourth breath, let the life force fill the head and neck as you exhale.

- With the fifth breath, let the life force fill all the organs of the belly as you exhale.

- With the sixth breath, let the life force fill the chest and heart centre as you exhale.

- With the seventh breath, as you exhale let the life force fill your whole energy field, harmonizing and balancing the energies within it.

- Stay for a few moments in your state of harmony and alertness.

You can vary how you direct the seven breaths according to your needs on any particular day. For example, you may need to focus more energy on a specific part of the body.

If you are able to do the exercise outside, notice the world around you as you calmly take your breaths. Feel your sacred connection with life being renewed. Acknowledge the other life forms that are present.

We are one with the sun and fire. Their life is our life.

We are one with air. Its life is our life. The state of air on the planet reflects the state of human thought. Every time that we work with air in a sacred manner (such as conscious breathing), we do something to bring harmony to human thinking and to return purity to the air.

SACRED MINDFULNESS – A CORE PRACTICE OF SPIRITUAL HEALING

Before starting work, healers consciously seek to link with the source of healing energies through a process of attunement (as described in more detail in Chapter 6, Preparing Sacred Space, for example). This book emphasizes that healing, at some level, will occur as the natural outcome of aligning ourselves with the sacred. As our healing practice was evolving, therefore, we have sought a method of spiritual alignment that attunes us to the Source on a more permanent basis, as a way of being. This is a form of meditation we call Sacred Mindfulness, which has become a core practice of Spiritual Healing. The Seven Breaths of Greeting described in Action Point 5 is an excellent preparation for the morning practice.

You may find it helpful to be familiar with Chapter 9 of *Your Healing Power*, which looks at meditation, but creating communion with Oneness does not depend on your previous knowledge or experience of meditation. Sacred Mindfulness is a way of being consciously centred, while totally alert and aware of the body and the outside world, as well as the subtle level of the heart centre and the soul. It is being mindful of the sacred within and without. This enables healing consciousness to be accessed at any time.

Practice induces a calming and eventual cessation of unnecessary mental activity. Breathing rate and heartbeat become calmer and slower. This may release unprocessed energies that have either been stored in the physical body or at the level of the emotions or mind. This is a normal and natural outcome of the healing that begins as soon as the link with soul consciousness is made. We have found that the calming and healing effects of Sacred Mindfulness practice combat stress and energize the body systems.

Establishing a pattern of practice

In the early stages of practice, it is very helpful to establish a pattern of time, place and position, which tells your mind and body that this is your appointment with the Source, your tryst with the Beloved, your communion with Soul. Notice how your mind reacts to this and what tricks it plays to get you to miss your appointment!

Early mornings and evenings are generally times when the world around us is most tranquil. These are times of stillness to which birds, especially, are sensitive. But choose a time which fits your lifestyle. If necesary, you are going to have to make time for your practice – 15 minutes twice a day.

If possible, set aside a special place that is clean and fresh. You might like to keep certain things in this place to remind you of what your practice is for. Choose a quiet, comfortable spot where you will not be disturbed.

Sit on the ground, or in a chair. It is most important to be comfortable, with the back and neck straight, but not tense or tight, and the hands resting on the thighs. If sitting in a chair, the feet should be flat on the floor. Relax the shoulders and hold the head erect. This position is known as 'sitting like a mountain'. You are solid, relaxed and calm, and your body is well connected with the ground with your head reaching to the sky.

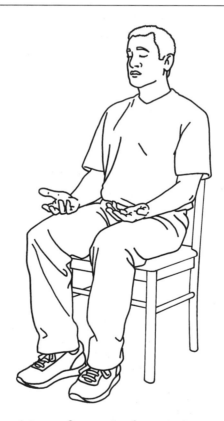

Figure 2. The sitting position – for use in the exercises and when sitting for visualization or meditation when the sensitivity of the palms is needed.

Sacred Mindfulness is not about leaving the world, but about being with, or in Oneness. We may acknowledge intellectually that we are one with all that is, but this is not our *experience* unless we make a conscious effort. Practice allows us to realize that Oneness is part of us; we are not separate from any other being or thing and Oneness is what we are.

Once this state is recognized it can be achieved when still or in motion, in the act of doing something or being somewhere other than your practice place. It is a state of consciousness that simply needs to be practised. Your attitude to this exercise is crucial. If it is a chore, change your attitude. See it like being with someone you dearly love – being with someone you love cannot be a chore, it is something to look forward to.

To establish a firm, grounded foundation for practice it is important to recognize the role of the body, and to create a relaxed and aware rapport with your body before moving into the deeper phases of the practice. This is how we begin:

ACTION POINT 6 Sacred Mindfulness Practice – Rapport with the Body

First part of core developmental tool – promoting awareness of the body as a vehicle of the sacred. Enhancing relationship with the physical body.

This exercise may also be used as a self-healing activity to improve relationship with the physical body. Its energizing potential helps to combat the harmful effects of stress.

- Sit in the position described above. Check that you are sitting straight and feeling balanced. Relax your body, especially the neck. As you relax, feel the shoulders and the hips sinking down.

- Use the breath to help you relax. As you breathe out, let go and relax. If you are aware of any worries or anxieties within, let go of them as you breathe out through the open mouth. Close the mouth once you feel settled.

- Allow the mind to gently follow the rhythm of your breath as you breathe in and then out.

- Now bring the mind to the heart energy centre in the centre of your chest. This is where soul resides. Let your attention rest there as you continue to follow your gentle breathing. Keep breathing into the heart centre. Be with your heart centre for a few moments.

- Slowly move your focus to the top of your head. Allow yourself to be aware of any sensations there. Let these sensations pass through your awareness. Rest in this awareness for some moments.

- Slowly let your attention move down your face, again allowing yourself to be aware of any sensations and letting them pass through your awareness. Rest in this awareness.

- Become aware of the back of your head, being aware of any sensations there and letting them pass through your awareness. Rest in this awareness.

- Slowly move your awareness to the throat and neck, across each shoulder and down each arm to each hand; down the front of your body; down your back; across the buttocks and pelvis; down each leg to each foot.

- This scanning awareness should be done very slowly and deliberately, giving yourself time to be aware of every part of your body and resting in your awareness at each stage.

- Once you reach your toes, make your way back up each leg; up the body; up each arm until you have returned to the top of your head, resting in your awareness as before.

- Now allow your awareness to trickle like water from the top of your head, over your whole body until you are aware of your whole body. Watch the passage of sensations and feelings as they pass through your awareness. Accept them all without judgement and without holding on to them. Rest in this non-grasping awareness.

- Continue to breathe gently into the heart centre as you allow any thoughts or emotions to come into and pass through your awareness. Keep checking that your body is relaxed. Note the content of mental or emotional material without engaging with it. Rest in your awareness.

- If the mind begins to intrude, focus on your heart centre breath and relax into your body's sensations.

In the beginning of this practice, you will be aware of yourself as witness to the sensations of your body. Later this will merge so that both you and the sensations are one. At this point, identification with your personality ceases, leaving a state of calm clarity.

When you have spent enough time practising mindfulness of the body so that you can reach a total, comfortable and relaxed awareness of it, you are ready to move to the second stage of Sacred Mindfuness. This brings mental peace, allowing a clear link with soul consciousness. The deeper levels of practice bring you to a state where there is no separation between you and soul consciousness.

The mind, when undisturbed by its programmes and our emotional reactions, returns to its pristine state. This enables us to have a deeper experience of Love and Peace. Free from distracting thoughts, we can enter the deep silence; we have a sense of internal clarity; we feel open, relaxed and accepting, not grasping at anything or trying to hold on to something.

When the mind reaches this harmonious state, thoughts may arise but they do not interfere with the clarity and harmony; they pass through our awareness. We become more open-hearted and willing to be consciously present in the now, not lingering in, hankering after or worrying about the past or the future.

ACTION POINT 7 Sacred Mindfulness – Deeper Practice – Rapport with the Mind and Emotions

Second part of core developmental tool – enhancing ability to expose mind and emotions to the light of soul.

This exercise may also be used in self- healing to monitor the activities of mind and emotions.

- Sit as before and allow yourself to reach a state of bodily relaxation as in Action Point 6 – the first stage of Sacred Mindfulness.

- Breathe into the heart centre and focus on the movement of your breath in and out of the heart centre. As soon as you find your awareness attaching itself to thoughts, bring it back to your rhythm of breathing into the heart centre.

- Keep to this level of awareness until you find that you can maintain it for 15 minutes at a time with your body relaxed.

- Having reached this stage, allow your attention to notice the passing of thoughts, images and sensations through your mind, without engaging with them. Notice how thoughts arise, pass through and disappear.

- As a thought disappears you can, for a moment, experience the clear mind state before the next thought appears. Rest in those moments of clarity.

- Proceed in the same way with any emotions or feelings that arise. Allow them to pass through your awareness without engaging with them.

- Allow yourself to be with soul in the silence of the heart centre. Enjoy the silence, the calm and the comfort of being with soul, then being Oneness.

- If you find you have moved away from your focus, bring it back by continuing to breathe into the heart centre. Being in this place of sacred silence is being mindful.

Stay with each part of the practice long enough for a feeling of relaxation and confidence to thoroughly ground it.

As you move deeper into the practice, your breathing and heartbeat blend with the intuitive flow of energy that is moving down into the heart centre. You may be aware of this flow in different ways – as colour, impressions or as feelings, for example. Realize that this awareness is a sign of your consciousness moving away from separation towards the experience of Oneness. The less you engage with your awareness, the further you will enter into the silence. Simply allow the intuitive energy to flow as it will, while you keep to your centre of silence. You may wish to record your awarenesses in your journal later.

Sacred Mindfulness opens up the channel to soul and we are made aware of what is clogging it – our inability to relate to the body; inability to relate to the planet; inability to relate to the natural world; inability to consciously choose our emotional state; inability to consciously choose our mental state. Gradually all these aspects of self are brought into harmony.

True practice means being diligent and dedicated without striving, forcing, wanting or grasping. The emphasis is on being. Sacred Mindfulness is a step-by-step way to being who we really are. It is no coincidence that this should be a healing state!

In time, show yourself that your practice is not confined to a specific place or to specific conditions. Sacred Mindfulness helps to heal the Earth. Reawaken your links with the natural world of the Earth and the Earth family by getting out into nature and practising there. The whole Earth family appreciates your light.

Finally, there are three sacred principles that will energize your practice of Sacred Mindfulness. These are:

1. Begin your practice from the heart, doing it because of Oneness – raising your consciousness raises all consciousness, pouring healing out into the cosmos.
2. Our inner eye knows that we do not need anything so we do not need to grasp at the practice – it is simply a way of being who we really are.
3. The practice has life force when it is offered to all beings as a gift. Close your practice by dedicating it to peace and harmony in the world.

By making sure that these three loving attitudes are in place, your practice has healing power.

FEEDING THE STOCK

When Jack worked on a farm, the rule was to feed the stock before feeding yourself. It is a rule we have tried to keep to whether we were living in town or country.

If you have carried out the above exercises before eating, now is a good time to think about 'feeding the stock'. Feed the birds in your garden and any animals in your care. This is a simple way to remember the animals and birds of the Earth family and our oneness with them. Following this we can recall, with thanks, our oneness with food, the food producers and the food sellers.

THE SACRED PATH TO INNER PEACE

Creating a way of being that will enhance our development as healers is an adventure in creativity. Use your imagination to find ways to support your practice. Entering the sacred silence of Oneness is difficult if we are in a turmoil about something. Whatever our physical, emotional or mental state, this is what we offer our patients, and these are the energies we radiate out into the world.

One of the most powerful forms of love we can generate is peace. Peace begins inside each one of us and an essential support to practice is a state of inner peace.

With this in mind, we have adapted the peace walk of the Iroquois as a creative way for healers. (The North American Iroquois Confederacy of Five Nations was formed in about 1570. The US Constitution and Bill of Rights was later modelled on the Confederacy principles of mutual welfare and security.) The sacred path to inner peace has seven places. You can remind yourself about this when you take your seven breaths in the morning or when you consider the seven energy centres of your etheric body, as described in Chapter 8.

Through the seven places, soul tells us about our journey as healers. Each place is a way of being and describes a certain attitude to life, ourselves and the Source. Once you have consolidated the first place, the next one builds upon it. Take time to allow this to happen, since each place on the path is dependent on all the others.

The seven places on the path to inner peace are:

- faith
- love
- awareness of soul contact
- awareness of the life force
- living creatively
- the hollow bone
- being in inner peace.

Faith

Soul has faith in life; that is why we come here. But we need to realize that there is enough of everything, including the resources for our needs. There is enough love. Soul cannot fail, it will succeed in carrying out its purpose. There are no exceptions to this.

Love

We have faith that the sun will always shine and it does. It sustains life on Earth and is a symbol of the light and warmth of the cosmic sun. We can see it is a symbol of the love of the Source. We will become aware of the love in Creation when we begin to love Creation. Soul comes here because it has faith in the love of the Source. The sun shines on all, showing us that true love is unconditional.

Awareness of soul contact

We all have intuition. This is our contact with soul. Intuition allows us to know that faith and love are real. Intuition tells us that there is no separation between anything, only Oneness. Our intuitive knowing means that we will have to revise our attitudes about judgement and condemnation of ourself and of others.

Awareness of the life force

All life is part of us. There is an energetic force that supports all life. This is the life force, which is another aspect of love. You felt this aspect of love when you carried out the Seven Breaths of Greeting in Action Point 5. When we see the green shoots of new plant growth, giving the promise of rebirth and regeneration, we are reminded again of the force of life.

Living creatively

This place on the sacred path to inner peace arises from awareness of the life force. Just as the natural world constantly reminds us of new creation, we understand that to be part of life is to live creatively. The previous four places showed us the presence of the God within. In creativity we practise being the God within. One of soul's most powerful ways of being creative is in healing.

The hollow bone

The sixth place draws our attention to the channel of our creativity, the hollow bone. How open and clear is it for what soul needs to express? How pure is our intention and what is our relationship with truth? How close are we to being authentic and what may be blocking the creative flow?

Being in inner peace

The seventh place on the sacred path to inner peace allays any anxiety we may have about our hollow bone. Here we can find all the previous places in life itself if we stop to look. The rainbow serves as a beautiful symbol of the protection and reassurance offered by the place of inner peace.

Soul is here. There *is* love and there is no separation. There is a way of contacting love. There is a life force that displays the power of love in the world around us. We can realize we are one with this love through our own power to love, imagine and create.

It is our decision about how the channel for our creativity will be used. There are no expectations and there will be no judgement or condemnation about what we decide to do. The seventh place tells us that we can enter the inner silence and experience the peace of Oneness. This is the birthright of all humans.

The sacred path to inner peace assures us that being at one with our true self is more important than any stress or anxiety we might have. If such things are in your way, use the breath and relaxation to bring harmony as you retrace your steps on the path and consolidate them again in your mind. Allow your Sacred Mindfulness practice to accompany you. Working with the path like this will help you to restore healing consciousness.

NOURISHMENT

Inner peace satisfies a soul need and becomes a form of nourishment. All aspects of our being need nourishing so that, as we progress in our work as healers, it is essential to be aware, at all levels, of what our needs really are. For example, does the body still need the foods we habitually consume or have the body's needs changed? Do we ever ask what it needs and have we listened to its reply?

Similarly, the type of emotional and mental nourishment we need begins to change and there will probably be a need for more peace and quiet.

What we want is not always what we need. The heart's guidance may not accord with current taste, fashion, societal norms or other pressures. Soul is able to impress us with its needs so we should not be surprised when it chooses to do this at any time and in any situation, encouraging us to review our wants and needs.

CREATIVITY AND THE MOVEMENT OF CREATIVE ENERGIES

An essential nourishment for the healer is creativity. The fifth place on the sacred path to inner peace reminds us that we are soul and that soul is God expressing God. Our creative energy is the force generated in the sacral energy centre – just below the navel, opposite the sacral bones of the spine – which is also a centre of power and processor of vitality energy. The sacral centre is our womb of creativity and any suppression of its energies is a threat to health and well-being. (More detailed information about the sacral centre follows in Chapter 8, Seven Sacred Steps.) The psychoanalyst Otto Rank's clinical experience was that lack of creativity in patients resulted in depression and pessimism.

When we are creative, mind is notified of our creation as the energy moves up into the solar plexus centre. Here, our sense of who we are is strengthened by this centre's awareness of the special energy passing through. The heart centre monitors our creation and is aware of whether it is created in love. If so, the heart centre is uplifted since all true creativity is a release of love (as was the original Creation). Finally, it is the task of the throat centre to facilitate the expression of our creativity.

THE NECESSITY OF PLAY

From birth, our instinct is to play. This is our creative way of finding out about ourselves and our environment. Once the baby feels safe and secure, it moves its attention from the base centre (at the base of the spine) to the sacral. Here, it is put in touch with creative energies and begins to play, at all levels. Very often, the smiles, noises and cries of a baby are its experiments with play. If the baby does not feel safe and secure it may well need to spend more time consolidating the energies of the base centre so that play activity begins later.

Inability to play is considered an illness in psychological terms. The psychologist D.W. Winnicott, who made a study of the function of play in creativity, considered that individuals could only discover themselves through being creative. Further, the child or adult has to be able to play in order to be creative. Spiritual Healing sees creativity as love in the form of play, an essential expression of our true nature. This is why creativity is one of the quickest and easiest ways of linking with soul and thus a vital aspect of personal development for the healer. Play, fun and creativity have to be part of our way of being.

CLEARING, REGULATING AND PROTECTING THE ENERGY SYSTEM

While play and finding ways to be creative are essential to our growth and well-being as healers, so is the management of our own energy field (aura).

When healing consciousness is operational, the subtle energy centres (chakras) are more open than usual. This enables them to transmit the quantity and quality of energies required during the healing session and also to process various other subtle energies that are flowing, in a two-way motion, during healing transactions. But the healer may also be open energetically, outside of the healing session, simply because this is a function of being a sensitive and aware person. As we have shown in this chapter, in Spiritual Healing the healer is taking a number of measures to upgrade their own energy field in order to make the healing channel as clear and effective as possible. This means that the healer is inevitably open to absorb energies that are of a slower vibration than their own.

Compared with healing energies or the life force, for example, much of the energy radiated by humans is of a relatively heavy nature, and has been generated by human thought. Some of this heavy energy is in the universal energy field around us; some we absorb from other people; and some is transmitted to us via thought.

Just as Sacred Mindfulness is a core practice in Spiritual Healing, management of the healer's energy field involves an essential support routine that has to be carried out every day. Looking after your 'hollow bone' is part of your responsibility to yourself and to Oneness. Here are the three support exercises you will need:

ACTION POINT 8 Clearing the Energy Field

Action Points 8, 9 and 10 are developmental tools for increasing awareness of our own energy field and energy centres. They may also be used as self-healing techniques, promoting awareness of the subtle energy system, and its need for clearing and protection.

At the end of the day, or whenever you are aware of the build-up of heavy energy, clear your energy field. This exercise may be carried out in a sitting position, where necessary.

- Stand with the feet a shoulder-width apart and your arms hanging loosely. Flex the knees to allow the body to relax. Use the breath to bring calmness and a feeling of being centred.

- Let yourself be aware of the heavy energy in your body and energy field. Notice where it seems to have accumulated or where it seems most prevalent. (Later, it is worth keeping a note of this observation in your journal to see if there is any pattern.)

● Now visualize yourself under a shower or gentle waterfall of silver light. Let this light pour over you, through you and out into your surrounding energy field, especially where you sensed an accumulation of heavy energy. Let it clear you inside and out. Allow the light to exit through the hands and feet and every orifice.

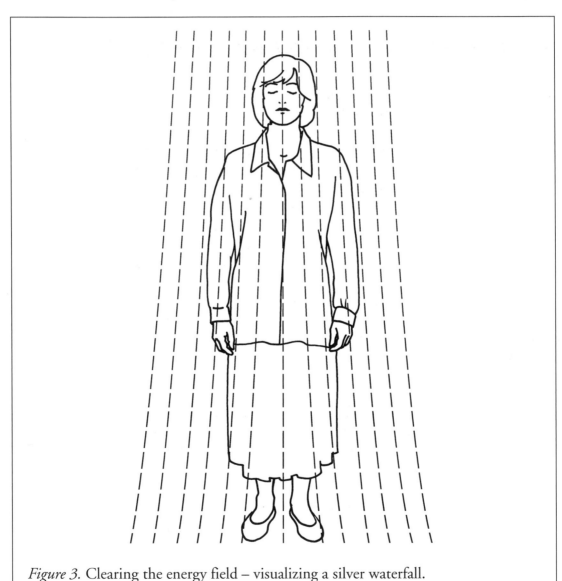

Figure 3. Clearing the energy field – visualizing a silver waterfall.

- Notice the colour of the light that tends to move in to replace the heavy energy you have cleared. Your awareness of this will confirm that the clearing is taking place.

Maintain this position and follow with the next exercise.

ACTION POINT 9 Regulating the Energy Centres

Promotes knowledge of our own energy centres and how they are affected by any spiritual activity.

See also note to Action Point 8. At the end of the day, or after activities such as healing, prayer, meditation, even reading related books, the energy centres are more open than usual, as described above. When not engaged in spiritual activities, the centres need to be returned to everyday functioning.

The structure of a centre may be visualized as a flower that is fully open, but now needs to close up a little. In the following exercise, do not allow any of the centres to completely close or they would, over time, stop functioning altogether.

See if you are aware of any centres that seem to be more open than others. Keep a note of this in your journal to see if there is any pattern or correlation between what you have been doing and the state of your energy centres. (Detailed information about the centres follows in Chapter 8, Seven Sacred Steps.)

- Following the clearing exercise, put your mind in the crown centre, at the top of the skull. If you find it helpful, think of its colour vibration as a violet light. Keep relaxed and breathing normally. Allow it to close up a little to process a lower ratio of energy transaction.

- Move your focus to the brow centre, in the centre of the forehead above the eyebrows. It has a royal blue or indigo light. Allow it to return to a lower ratio of functioning.

- Move to the throat centre. It has a sky blue light. Allow it to return to a lower ratio of functioning.

- Move to the heart centre, in the centre of your chest. It has a green light. Allow it to return to a lower ratio of functioning.

- Move to the solar plexus centre, just below the diaphragm and above the navel. It has a golden yellow light. Allow it to return to a lower ratio of functioning.

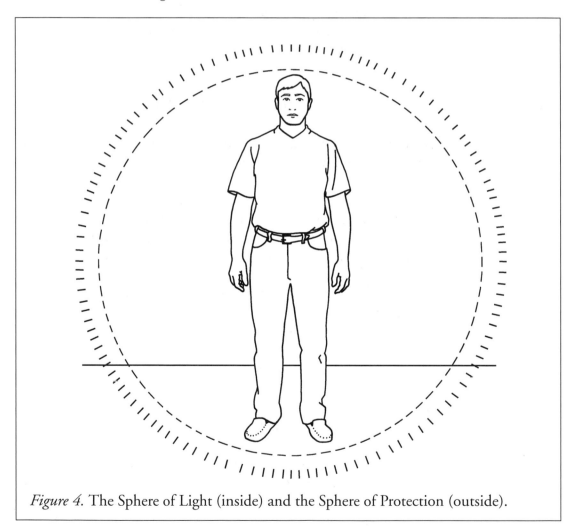

Figure 4. The Sphere of Light (inside) and the Sphere of Protection (outside).

- Move to the sacral centre, below the navel and opposite the sacral bones of the spine. It has an orange light. Allow it to return to a lower ratio of functioning.

- Move to the base centre at the base of the spine. It has a red light. Allow it to return to a lower ratio of functioning.

- You now need to surround yourself with a sphere of light. The first colour that comes to mind is the colour of light which will keep your system intact. See the sphere of coloured light totally surrounding you.

Follow with the next exercise.

ACTION POINT 10 Protecting the Energy Field

The final part of the closing down routine keeps your energy field strong and will not allow the entry of incompatible energies.

This exercise should be used at the end of the day and at any other time when you feel the need to look after your personal field, such as when travelling, going shopping or being with crowds of people or individuals whose energies seem incompatible with your own.

- Still relaxed and breathing normally, surround your sphere of coloured light with a sphere of golden light (Figure 4). See it sparkle, flash and gleam. This tells you about its energy of strength and protection. Spend a moment of awareness before moving into other activities.

REVIEWING THE DAY

The purpose of looking back over your day is not about self-judgement or self-condemnation, but it is about self-discovery. This happens through bypassing the mind (the part of us that makes judgements in the light of conditioning) by getting in touch with soul.

ACTION POINT 11 Recalling Soul Communication

Developmental tool — increases ability to communicate with soul and to practise being present to soul.

Used on a regular basis, this exercise is a self-healing technique for enhancing soul communication.

In this exercise we are seeking communication with soul. You may need to keep a notebook and writing materials handy.

- At the end of the day, sit or lie comfortably and relax the body. Use the breath to bring calm and balance to the mind.

- Let your focus move gently to the heart centre where soul resides. Make the request to soul, 'What have you been saying to me today?'.

- Wait patiently for soul's reply. It may well come in picture form, like watching a video. There may be a replay of the day's happenings or other visual images that relate to them. Be open for soul's surprises.

- If you feel the need to make a note of anything, do it now. You may have forgotten it by tomorrow.

As explained above, you will soon be able to tell if your communication is from soul. Its tone will be loving and accepting, not judgemental or condemning.

Since this exercise may open up your energy centres, it should be carried out before the closing down procedure described in the previous exercises (Action Points 9 & 10).

You now have in place the most important activities that you are going to need to maintain your integrity as a healer — these are prayer, meditation and clearing your energy field. Regulating the subtle energy system and protecting your field should be seen as sealing the clearing work, when this is appropriate.

Having established a way of being that supports your practice, you are ready to work with the healing consciousness. In the next chapter we look at how to prepare yourself and the healing space to do this.

6

Preparing Sacred Space

There is no such person as a 'patient' until they meet the caring or healing agent. And there is no such person as the 'carer' or 'healer' until they meet the person who seeks their help, the patient. So it is in the sacred meeting that they become what they are, see what they may be, or perhaps realize what they are not. The truth of this, arising out of Oneness, reminds us not that patients are inferior to us, but that we are not superior to them.

The purpose of preparation, then, is to celebrate the meeting of souls. The method is to attain a consciousness that is attuned to soul and to create a meeting place that is most appropriate to the joyous occasion. This chapter suggests ways in which we can be sure about this.

It was Barry's first afternoon as a therapist at the complementary health centre. As he walked into the reception room, he was immediately alerted to a change in energy that contrasted with the tree-lined avenue outside. The atmosphere felt heavy, he experienced it in his heart centre. His hands started tingling – his healing signal. What was going on? He hadn't started working, yet something needed healing. He sensed that the room was filled with the energy traces of the morning's patients.

Barry set about protecting himself and then clearing his practice room. As he sat to prepare the sacred space, he discovered that there was more than patients' energies to clear, it seemed that the building itself needed clearing and healing. After this he put a sphere of protective light around the building. Only then did he feel that he was ready for his patients. This reminded Barry that incompatible energies may be present, not only in the spaces of the rooms, but in the walls and fabric of a building.

Barry resolved to raise the issue of energy hygiene at the next therapists' meeting. This would ensure a healthier environment for the patients to enter, and for the therapists and reception staff to work in. If they wished, he would also teach the therapists about protecting their own energy fields and clearing the energy in their practice rooms at the end of every day.

CREATING AWARENESS

With Barry's experiences in mind, we can begin by looking at the general state of our sensitivity and awareness. This is a simple and enjoyable first step in developing the consciousness needed to work intuitively with the subtle energies of healing.

ACTION POINT 12 Awareness of the Personal Energy Field

Development tool – promoting sensitivity to one's own subtle energy field.

Action Points 12 and 13 may also be used as self-healing activities promoting awareness of internal and external subtle energies.

- Sit comfortably with your feet flat on the floor and with your hands, palms down, resting on the thighs. Be aware of your feet in contact with the ground. Take three full breaths and relax the body, especially the neck, shoulders and elbows.

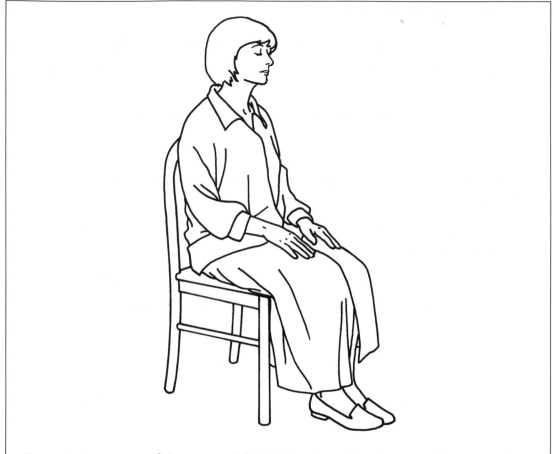

Figure 5. Awareness of the personal field. Note the palms down position.

- Allow yourself to be at one with your body and the energy field that permeates and surrounds it. What is your first impression of the energies within yourself? Are there light and dark areas. Do they relate to how you feel today?

- Now allow yourself to merge more deeply with the energies inside. Take your time. What is your awareness now?

- Turn your hands palms up. Let your focus move out into the personal field that surrounds your physical body. What are you aware of?

- Make a note of your impressions.

Stand up and move around for a few moments before carrying out the next awareness exercise.

ACTION POINT 13 Awareness of the Energies Outside the Personal Field

Developmental tool – increasing sensitivity to external subtle energies.

- Sit comfortably as in the previous exercise. This time position your hands with the palms up. (**Note**: Keeping the hands palms up at any time ensures that you will be open to absorb energy or energetic information through the energy centres of the palms. In some exercises this can be helpful, while in some exercises it can be otherwise, so use your intuition to decide how you wish to position the hands.)

- What is your first impression of the room's energies?

- Allow your own energies to merge with the room. What do you pick up now?

- Feel your energy centres open and aware, including those of the hands and feet. Allow the energies of the room to impact on each centre. Start with the feet, then the base, sacral, solar plexus, heart, hands, throat, brow and crown. What is your awareness of the way the room impacts on your centres?

- Make your journal notes as necessary.

ATTUNEMENT OF SELF

From awareness of self and the surroundings, we move to consciously re-creating the energy patterns of the self and the surroundings as the next step in preparation of sacred space.

69

The daily practice of Sacred Mindfulness builds a consciousness that can instantly move into healing mode. While this healing consciousness is being developed, it is helpful to practise other exercises that will strengthen our links with the source of healing energies.

These exercises are ways of attuning the mind, emotions and body to the 'voice' of soul. This means that we are signalling to soul that we are ready to hear, that it can speak and we are ready to listen.

This is how a healer can operate straight away when they are needed, especially in an emergency, because attunement and centring practice is constantly signalling to soul that the healer is ready to listen to soul guidance. There is an ear of attention and an ear of intention that may be linked to any or all of the senses.

To open the listening ear of attunement, first make sure you have cleared your field of heavy energy by carrying out Action Point 8 – Clearing the Energy Field. You can now bring your field into energetic balance by carrying out the Rainbow Breath:

ACTION POINT 14 The Rainbow Breath

Promoting energetic balance within the subtle energy system. Working with the breath and the colours of the seven main energy centres.

This exercise may also be used as a self-healing strategy for clearing and rebalancing the subtle energy field.

- Stand, or sit if necessary, with your feet a shoulder-width apart. Let the arms hang loosely by your sides. Relax the body.

- Take a few breaths to clear the lungs. Allow any tension, worry or anxieties to exit as you exhale through the open mouth. Close the mouth and breathe normally when you feel settled.

- You are now going to fill your energy field with seven spheres of coloured light, from red to violet. Each sphere should be visualized as outside of the one you created before.

- Breathe in, visualizing red light rising from behind your heels, moving up your back to the top of your head. Pause for a moment.

- As you exhale, visualize the red light moving down the front of your body until it is under your feet. You are now enclosed in a sphere of red light.

- Breathe up orange light and surround the red sphere with it, making sure that it totally encloses the sphere of red light and creates an orange sphere outside it.

- Breathe up golden yellow light and surround the orange sphere.

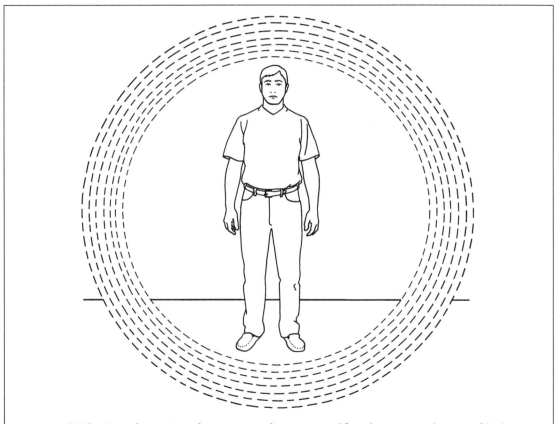

Figure 6. The Rainbow Breath – surounding yourself with seven spheres of light to clear and balance the energy field.

- Breathe up green light and surround the golden yellow sphere.

- Breathe up sky blue light and surround the green sphere.

- Breathe up royal blue/indigo light and surround the sky blue sphere.

- Breathe up violet/purple light and surround the royal blue sphere.

- Spend a few moments of awareness as you are totally enclosed in a rainbow of light.

Then move on to the next exercise.

ACTION POINT 15 Attunement of Self

Developmental tool – alignment with soul, necessary for all healing activities.

The first three stages of this exercise may also be used as a self-healing technique to achieve a sense of being centred.

- Sit comfortably with your feet flat on the floor and with your hands, palms up, resting on the thighs (see Note in Action Point 13).

- Be aware of your feet in contact with the ground and aware that you are linking with the energies of the Earth, via your base centre, at the base of your spine. Take three full breaths and relax the body, especially the neck, shoulders and elbows.

- Be aware of your heart and crown centres opening and allow yourself to be at one with your soul. Spend a few moments in Oneness with your soul. Remind yourself that soul is at one with the Source.

- Give thanks to the Source for the opportunity to be used as a channel for healing. Ask to be as pure a channel as possible. Ask for protection for yourself and your patients. Dedicate yourself and your work and ask for it to be blessed. Add any other prayers you wish, aware that the Source is part of you.

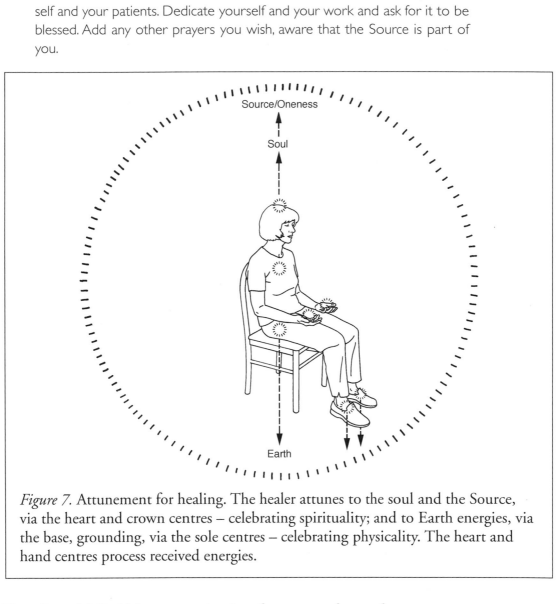

Figure 7. Attunement for healing. The healer attunes to the soul and the Source, via the heart and crown centres – celebrating spirituality; and to Earth energies, via the base, grounding, via the sole centres – celebrating physicality. The heart and hand centres process received energies.

Your Sacred Mindfulness practice is, of course, a form of attunement. Through conscious attunement you have made your link with your soul and the source of healing energies. In doing so you have activated the first side of the Healing Triangle (in the following illustration, the triangle is set

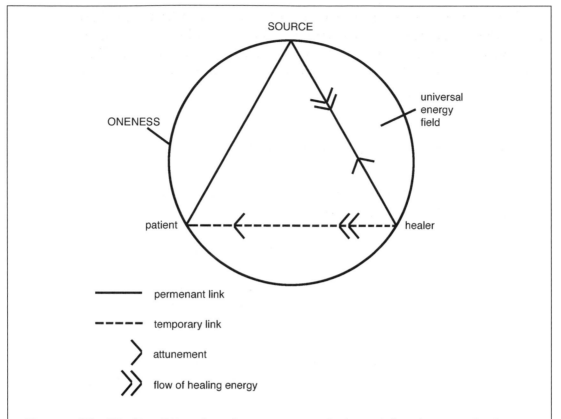

Figure 8. The Healing Triangle – showing energy links and flow between healer, patient and the Source of healing energies.

within a circle to signify the oneness of all three points). When you link with the soul of the patient (or a person to whom you are sending distant healing) you activate the second side. This, in turn, opens up the patient's link with the Source, activating the third side of the Healing Triangle.

ATTUNEMENT OF THE HEALING SPACE

You are preparing the working place for the Source to enter in. First, pay attention to the physical aspects of the space. It should be clean and all wastebins emptied. Flowers and drinking water should be fresh.

Next, clear the room of any heavy energies, as you did with yourself. This can be done with smoke, such as incense. Some healers like to use sound, such as a bell or clapping the hands. It is traditional in native Canadian West Coast healing to use a light source, such as a candle. Your intention is what is guiding the clearing process.

ACTION POINT 16 Preparing the Healing Space

Developmental tool – addressing the subtle energies of place. Creating a balanced energy field in which to work.

This technique may also be used to clear personal living space, promoting a healthy energetic environment.

If you have not had time to carry out the Attunement of Self exercise (Action Point 15), you can incorporate it into preparing the work place as in the first step below:

- Light an incense stick. Dedicate the light to the Light. Ask for protection as you open yourself up to be a channel for healing energies. Ask for help to be as pure a channel as possible.

- If you have already attuned, through Sacred Mindfulness practice or by the exercise Attunement of Self above, dedicate the smoke of the incense and ask that it may be used to clear, balance and harmonize the work place.

- Remain centred as you hold the incense stick and intuitively face a certain direction of the space. Move in a circle from where you are standing, allowing the smoke to spread out into the space before you. Take your time and do not hurry this procedure.

- If you find you need to move in an anticlockwise direction, you are clearing the energies of the space. If you find you need to move in a clockwise/sunwise direction, you are filling the space with new energies.

- As you move round you might like to ask that the space be cleared of all energies that are not compatible with healing. Ask that the space be filled with the energies of healing – the energies of Peace, Love and Light. Ask for a blessing on the space and all who enter it, and that they may benefit from the energies of Peace, Love and Light.

- If you work in a building shared by others, ask for a blessing on the room, the building and all who work (and live) in it, and that they may benefit from the healing energies.

- Wait for an intuitive signal that the job of clearing and preparing the space has been completed. If this is not forthcoming, wait to be given, intuitively, your next instruction.

This is how the room may be attuned to become sacred space. The room is of course conscious, but attunement raises this consciousness by accelerating the vibration of energy in the room in the same way as it raises the vibration of the healer's energy field.

After completion of the day's work, thank the space and clear (energetically) the furniture you have used – the healing couch, chairs, etc. Leave the room how you would wish to find it. This is your gift to the other therapists who share the room with you, or to yourself for the following day.

The clearing, preparation and attunement exercises help to create harmony at all levels of our being and within the work space.

Much of the energetic activity of attunement occurs on a subtle level, involving energies that vibrate faster than the speed of light. Recall that we have a subtle energy system that processes these energies, the energies of healing and the other subtle energies that are vital to our lives as physical, emotional, mental and spiritual beings. This is known as the Etheric Body, a modified form of soul's original Light Body.

The Soul
Systems

7

The Light Body

'Our God is Light. A day will come when you will understand what this means.' Pierre Bonnard

Soul first had contact with planet Earth through an energy pattern, which may be envisaged as a body of light. 'Light', in the sense generally used in this book, refers to an energy frequency greatly beyond the speed of physical light and is another term for 'spirit' – the energy of the Source. But the complete *experience* of physicality, existence on Earth and the tremendous pull of gravity, needs the denser energy form of the physical body. Choosing to incarnate into a physical body is what being human is about.

Because of the vast difference between the frequencies of the light body and the physical, an energetic bridging level was created by modifying the energies and structure of the light body. This modified light form is what is known as the *etheric body*.

In this chapter, we show how the purpose of all spiritual healing modes is defined by the fact that we are souls with a physical body, not bodies with a soul. We will also point out the crucial role that the etheric body has played and continues to play in the wondrous expression of soul that we are.

Further, we will show that there is no understanding of healing without an understanding of the etheric structure and its processes.

SUBTLE ENERGIES – THE FIFTH FORCE?

Scientists have discovered four forces by which they try to explain all the observable phenomena of the known universe. These are the strong nuclear force (as in the nucleus of the atom), the weak nuclear force, electromagnetic force and gravitational force.

But there is a growing body of data, especially in the field of subtle energy medicine, which cannot be explained in terms of these four forces. This data needs the presence and action of what some scientists, such as William Tiller, call *subtle energies*, the fifth force. From the point of view of Spiritual Healing, subtle energies are those travelling beyond the speed of light, which are vital to life and are intimately involved in healing, health and well-being.

Interpreting subtle energies

The healer's first encounter with subtle energies is when they are sensed at an etheric level. The energetic information is passed, via the brow centre, to the brain. The brain interprets subtle energetic information as best it can by comparing it with the physical phenomena it has already experienced. Hence healers develop a range of ways of describing subtle energies and energetic effects, including colours, sounds, smells, feelings and sensations, and various other awarenesses. Within Spiritual Healing this range of interpretations is valid. The inability of technology to quantify subtle energy makes it difficult for many to accept its existence – even when they are aware of it themselves.

CHARACTERISTICS OF THE ETHERIC BODY

Vibrating at a frequency beyond the speed of light, the etheric body projects some 5 to 10cm beyond the edge of the physical body. Since its detection by western clairvoyants over a hundred years ago, little is understood about the etheric and its origins, and its fundamental importance to life and healing.

In practice, we have noticed that the etheric body has a shape somewhat

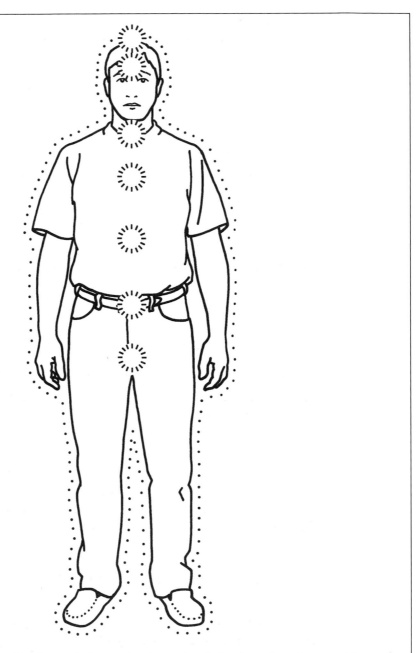

Figure 9. The physical body and the projecting etheric body – showing position of the seven main centres.

like the human form, with an outer surface composed of a glowing web-like structure, the whole appearing to be illuminated from within. The luminous depths contain hundreds of what look like even brighter lines of light, some running from the top to the base of the form. We have seen that the 'lines of light' are transparent channels, permitting the flow of a vast range of subtle energies, which appear as moving streams or threads of light. Where these channels cross each other, a node or vortex of light is formed. This makes looking at the etheric body very much like looking at the stars of the Milky Way.

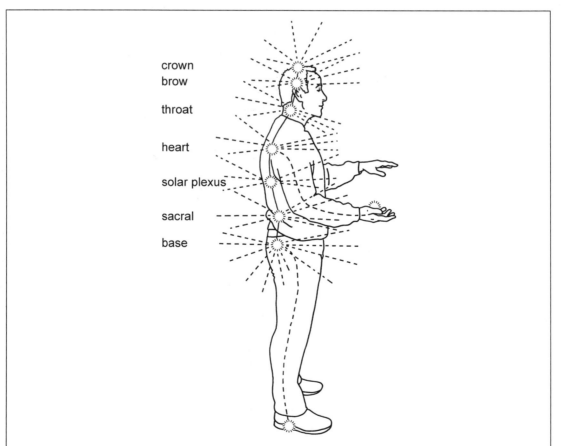

Figure 10. The seven main centres showing projection of energies – also palm and sole centres.

The nodes of light are the subtle energy centres (also known as *chakras*, from Sanskrit *chakram*, wheel) of the etheric body. The more channels that converge, the larger the centre and the more prominent are its activities. The larger centres are engaged in processing and monitoring energy flow. The seven main energy centres are seen to be connected to a central channel aligned with the spine. You will recall working with them already (as in Action Points 6, 7, 9, 11, 13 and 14, for example). We shall be describing the centres in more detail in Chapter 8, Seven Sacred Steps.

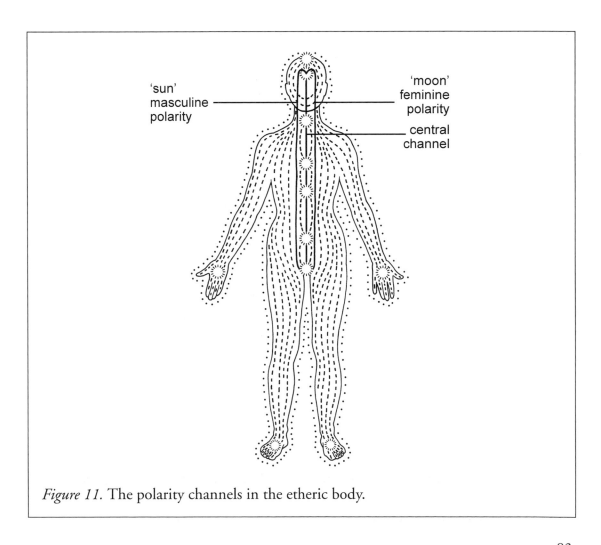

Figure 11. The polarity channels in the etheric body.

The polarity channels of the etheric body

On each side of the central channel, and connected to it, are two further channels, which extend from the base to the brow centres. The circulation of energy in the two channels creates a balance between the inflow and outflow of subtle energies throughout the system, including each of the centres. The polarities of energy are sometimes referred to as 'masculine' and 'feminine'. These classifications are historical and describe qualities of energy flow and not aspects of gender. The masculine, or emissive, right side of the field has energies that are outgoing. The feminine, or receptive, left side has energies that are incoming (Figure 11).

For emotional and mental health, as well as physical well-being, the energies of the two polarities need to be in a state of balance, but it is easy for them to get out of balance. For example, when we are not assertive enough and allow ourselves to be disempowered, the emissive energies are not being used when they need to be. The polarities are either thrown out of balance or their imbalance has caused us to be unable to stand up for ourselves.

When one energy stream is unused or underdeveloped, the other will try to compensate by dominating the system and all its activities. This is self-defeating since it nurtures the weakness.

In Sacred Healing, the healer notes whether healing is needed to bring polarity balance by working with the feet (as we shall see in the Healing Procedure in Chapter 14). This is later matched with the patient's story. When the story indicates that there could be a state of imbalance, a simple exercise can be used to empower the patient to see for themselves.

ACTION POINT 17 Checking Polarity Balance

Developmental tool – increasing awareness of balance within the human energy field.

This exercise needs a partner.

- Your partner should lie on a healing couch or sit in a chair. Ask your partner to use the breath to aid relaxation, and then breathe normally.

● Stand by your partner's feet, or opposite your seated partner and relax yourself too. Allow your relaxed gaze to scan your partner's body. Visualize it as luminous and transparent, like the etheric. See if you are aware of the same quality of light throughout the body. Are there darker areas? Keep a mental note.

● Now ask your partner to imagine being able to look inside their own body to see the quality of the light within. Then ask your partner to visualize a line dividing the body down the middle and to assess whether each half has the same quality of light. Are there any darker areas ?

● Compare your assessment with your partner's awareness.

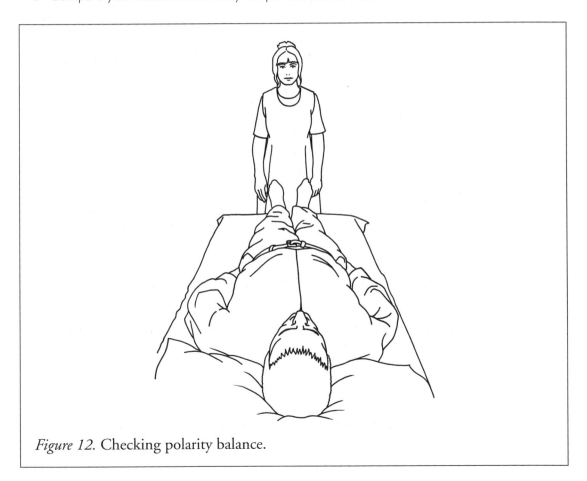

Figure 12. Checking polarity balance.

Your assessment can be followed with the next Action Point, which is how you would deliver balancing energies in the healing session (as described in The Sacred Meeting, Chapter 14).

ACTION POINT 18 Balancing Polarity

Developmental tool – practice in bringing energies into a harmonious state within the human energy field.

● Your partner should lie on the couch as before. You are standing by your

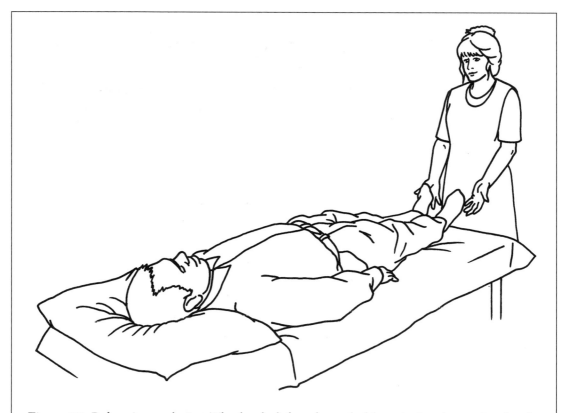

Figure 13. Balancing polarity. The healer's hands are held opposite the patient's sole centres.

partner's feet. If your partner is sitting in a chair, proceed in the same way, by squatting near your partner's feet.

- Hold your palms 5 to 10cm away from the soles (or tops) of the feet and allow the transfer of energy from yourself to your partner. Do not forget that in a healing session your own energies would not be involved because you would be chanelling the light.

- What do you notice and what is your partner aware of?

- After two to three minutes, ask your partner to look again into their body to reassess the balance of the light within. Is there any change?

THE PHYSICAL BODY IS A SOUL CREATION

The formation, development and composition of the physical body is controlled by the etheric. The etheric structures are the modifications made to the light body so that it can act as a template for the physical. For example, the symmetry of the physical body is derived from the symmetry of the etheric. The body's ability to process the flow of substances to and from the organs is derived from the flow of energies in the etheric polarity channels. The seven main energy centres are the structures from which the seven endocrine glands are derived. Other physical organs are derived from other large energy centres. The nervous system is derived from the system of etheric energy channels and the vascular (blood) system from the flow of energies within the etheric network. These foundations of the physical body have a direct bearing on how healing energies flow into it from a soul level.

Throughout the existence of the body, the etheric conveys the life force, essential to the animation of all physical forms, along with two vitalizing energies, which are conducted via the sacral and solar plexus centres.

In this way, the etheric is the energetic support system for physical life. The etheric level (of energy vibrations) is the gateway between the physical and the non-physical and, more importantly, the entry level for the light of soul into physical life. The healer follows this path by making contact first with the patient's etheric energy system.

The etheric facilitates the release of the soul from the physical and receives the soul during the first stage of death.

MENTAL AND EMOTIONAL SUBTLE ENERGIES

To facilitate life in the embodied, or human state, soul created mind as its instrument. Mind is therefore an aspect of soul consciousness that is entirely human. When mind interacts with physical life, feelings and emotions are generated. This creates a further aspect of soul consciousness, which, again, is entirely human.

The frequencies of mental and emotional energies are faster than the etheric so they radiate beyond this level. These energies occur in the human energy field as a series of zones (Figure 14).

The energetic pattern known as the 'emotional body' is that zone of energy vibration where emotional material, because of its frequency, is stored and/or processed. It should not be confused with the 'astral' vehicle, mentioned below.

The energetic pattern known as the 'mental body' is that zone of energy vibration where thought and mental material, because of its frequency, is stored and/or processed.

The term 'body' is in general use, but is quite misleading. Soul does not inhabit a separate mental body or a separate emotional body; rather these are complex zones of energy that arise as a direct result of soul's embodiment in the physical, through being human.

When we refer to the mental and emotional zones as 'levels' in this book, we are describing levels of energy frequency within the human energy field, the aura.

THE HUMAN ENERGY FIELD (AURA)

The human energy field may be visualized as a sphere of radiations that are the embodied energies of the soul. The densest, the physical, are at the centre, surrounded by the subtle energies of the etheric, emotional, mental, and soul levels. In the zone of soul energies, the slowest vibration gives a definition or boundary to the individual energy field.

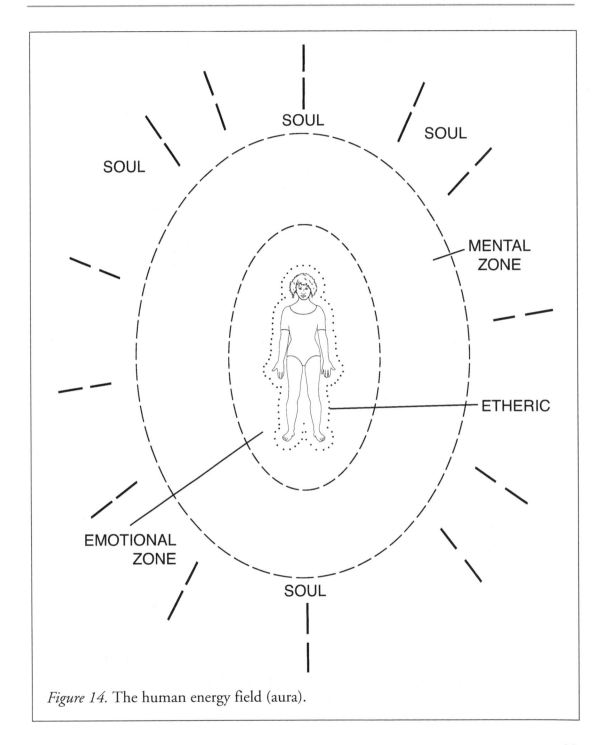

Figure 14. The human energy field (aura).

The 'astral' body

All the zones of energy have a range of vibration whose frequency bands are slowest at the 'edge' nearest the physical. The etheric body has a range of vibration that is slowest where it is close to the physical and faster where it is close to the so-called 'astral body'. This is the subtle energy vehicle used by soul to travel on levels *outside* the physical. (The astral body and its functions are described in more detail in Chapter 16, Distant Healing.)

In practice, we have observed how the centres link with all levels of the aura via energy channels that extend from the etheric to the 'defined edge' of the field. These energy channels are the link between the energies of the soul and the etheric, via the crown channel, and the link between the physical level, especially the planet, and the etheric, via the base channel (Figure 15). They play an important role in the healing procedure, as shall be pointed out later (in Chapter 14, The Sacred Meeting).

There is no actual division at the highest levels of soul energy between one 'soul' and another. All is spirit, all is Oneness. The reality of embodiment is that the energy of soul permeates and surrounds all levels of being.

Awareness of the aura

The aura (human energy field) contains evidence of the soul's experiences in its embodied form on earth. Intuitive and clairvoyant vision is able to detect this material. Such energetic information is often made available to healers.

We can be aware of the vibrations in our own field and we can also be aware of the energy fields of others, such as animals, plants and minerals, and the universal field that surrounds us.

Many are born with this awareness close to the surface. The poet William Wordsworth could recall his own awareness as a child:

There was a time when meadow, grove, and stream,
The earth and every common sight,
To me did seem
Apparelled in celestial light,
The glory and the freshness of a dream.

from *Intimations of immortality from recollections of early childhood* (1803)

In most people, these awarenesses are unconscious in daily life. But we are

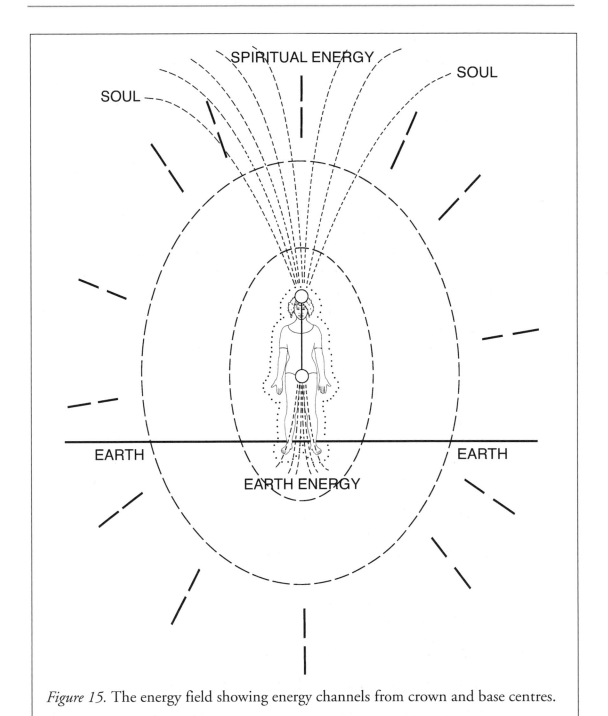

Figure 15. The energy field showing energy channels from crown and base centres.

conscious of them at some level of our being. Whether conscious or not, we are all equipped to process every level of energy, from the physical to soul.

In the following exercises you can begin to use your sensitivity to work with the energy field of another person.

ACTION POINT 19 Activating the Palm Centres

Developmental tool – to become familiar with the energetic structure of the hands.

Carried out before any sensing with the hands, this exercise may be used to prepare the energy centres of the palms to work at a subtle level.

- Close both hands to make a loose fist, squeezing the tips of the fingers against the palms. Do this a number of times in rapid succession until you feel intuitively that they are energized.

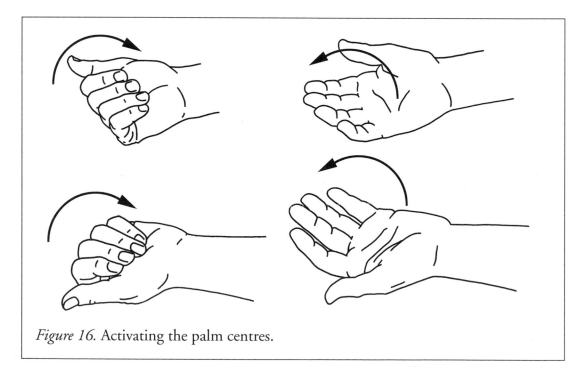

Figure 16. Activating the palm centres.

• The same result may be achieved by putting the palms together and gently rubbing them in a circular motion.

Now you are ready to carry out the next exercise.

ACTION POINT 20 Sensing the Human Energy Field

Developmental tool – using the energetic structure of the palms to sense the human energy field.

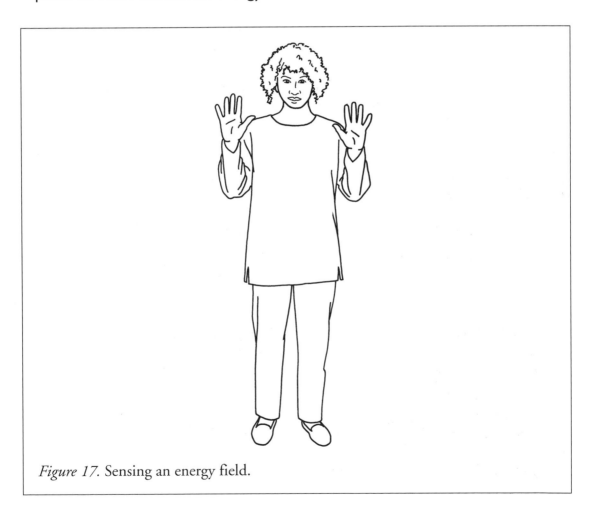

Figure 17. Sensing an energy field.

You will need to do this with a partner.

- First, see if you can locate your partner's field and sense its boundary. Ask your partner to stand in a relaxed position and to breathe normally without focusing on what you are doing. Stand a good ten paces away from your partner.

- Face your partner and hold your hands up in front of you with the palms facing your partner. Relax and breathe normally. Put your attention into your hands (Figure 17).

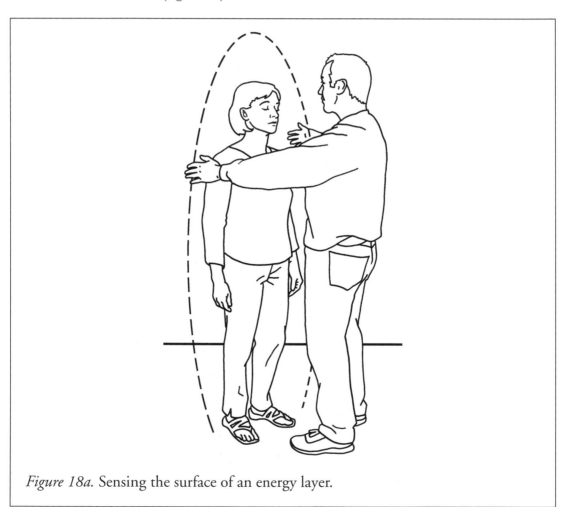

Figure 18a. Sensing the surface of an energy layer.

- Now walk towards your partner very slowly and stop when you feel you can sense the 'edge' of your partner's energy field. Allow yourself to fully sense this boundary through your hands.

- Assuming the field to be roughly spherical in shape, move round the 'outside' of the field, using the sensitivity of your palm centres to guide you. Move the hands upwards and downwards over the energetic 'surface' that you can sense. Try to move with the sensation you were first aware of. When you have completed your sensing, note the shape that you have actually defined (Figures 18a and 18b). Relax.

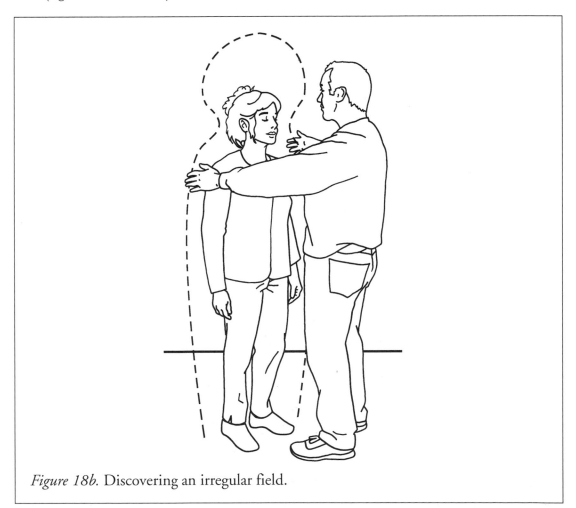

Figure 18b. Discovering an irregular field.

● Hold up your hands again, facing your partner. Now see if you can sense another 'layer' of energy in your partner's field as you move very slowly towards your partner. See how sensitive you are to the edge of this new energy zone. Move with this sensation only to see if you can make a second circuit around your partner. The more relaxed you are, the easier it will be to sense the energy levels.

● Hold your hands up towards your partner and proceed as before. Finally, decide how many zones of energy you sensed in your partner's field and where they seemed to be located. Note the shape they seemed to have.

● Talk about your experiences with your partner, then let your partner work on you. Compare notes.

Like most of the exercises in this book, this Action Point should be repeated from time to time. Each repetition increases your awareness and sensitivity.

Do not allow yourself to be influenced by what you *think* you ought to be aware of. The key to all sensing work is the element of fun! It is not a test. Your awarenesses are valid. Keep a note of your findings to build up your own database.

Take a break before working with the next Action Point.

ACTION POINT 21 Sensing Information in the Energy Field

Developmental tool – increasing awareness of subtle energy systems at work, giving and receiving subtle energetic information.

You will need to work with a partner. Remember the note on confidentiality in Chapter 2, Working With This Book.

● Sit opposite each other without touching. Both of you should relax and breathe normally. Your partner should be as passive as possible. You should both close your eyes to avoid absorbing information visually. The exercise should last from two to five minutes.

- As you sit opposite your partner, realize that their energy field includes the radiations of the mental and emotional subtle bodies. These contain mental and emotional material. Allow yourself to be open to this material and see if you become aware of it.

- Now consciously feel your energy centres being open to energetic information from your partner. What are you aware of this time?

- Relax and share your impressions with your partner. See if your partner agrees with your impressions or wants to comment on them.

- Have a short break before your partner works with you. Again, share and compare notes.

You have been working with the communication 'vehicles' of your partner. Since the energies stored in them become part of the energy field, they may be accessed through a simple attunement exercise like the Action Point described above.

THE COMMUNICATION VEHICLES OF THE HUMAN

The physical, mental and emotional bodies are the communication vehicles of the human. They communicate the experience of being human both to the person themselves and to the soul (via the subtle energy system of the etheric).

Through its structures, the etheric controls the energy that is made available to the physical, mental and emotional levels. This has important implications for healing, as we shall see.

THE COMMUNICATION VEHICLE OF THE SOUL

The etheric is the communication vehicle for the soul, reminding us that we are *more* than human and that humanness is just one part of our being. So that, while it is important for healers to know about and understand mind, emotions and the physical, it is far more important for them to know and understand the etheric and its structures and the progress of energy into, through and beyond the etheric. For this is the understanding of the energetic language of the soul.

PERSONALITY AND THE SOUL QUEST

As we saw in The Soul Journey, Chapter 3, through the interaction of the three human communication vehicles, a second 'self' emerges, the personality. From the point of view of the mind and emotions, this is the one who is having the experience of being human and who appears to be the only self. So when we identify with the personality alone, this is how we feel and spiritual reality seems far away, out of reach or actually unreal.

But our roots are in the spiritual and soul encourages us to find them through a wonderful variety of messages, including dreams, meetings with people and situations, encounters with animals and birds, synchronicities, even health conditions. The aim of the message is to open the way for the light to come back into our lives.

Sometimes we receive only part of the message and try to find our roots in life, through relationships, the family, community and culture. Some go on a quest to find their roots, or a pilgrimage to a sacred place, reflecting the human quest for reconciliation with soul. These great adventures, which Joseph Campbell called *The Hero's Journey*, are the stuff of myth and legend, stories and tales, full of difficulties and trials – just like our own lives.

SOUL COMMUNICATION

Soul communicates with the personality (what we think of as 'us') through the etheric. It is etheric consciousness that directs the soul message first to our mind, then the emotions, then the body. More often than not, our mind blocks the signal because of its conditioning. Similarly, it can suppress our emotional response. If this happens, the soul message is conveyed to the body where a physical condition or response is generated. This is how many of our aches and pains, accidents and incidents, are actually clues to an earlier soul message, which the mind and emotions have blocked, missed or suppressed.

Sacred Mindfuless practice (Action Points 6 and 7) helps us to gain a

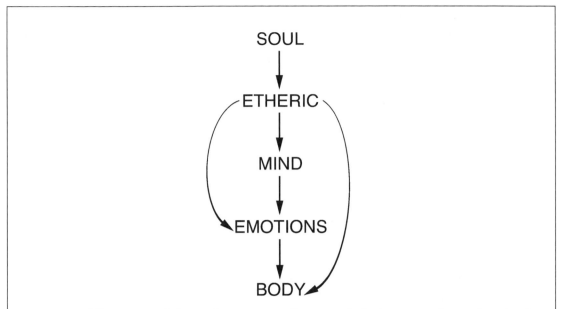

Figure 19. The route of the soul message – first to mind, then emotions, then body.

measure of control over such forms of mental interference, which can influence our effectiveness as people and as healers.

THE ETHERIC AND THE LIGHT

The etheric is the remnant of the original light body so that it has a close affinity with light and all other light bodies in the universe, such as the sun and stars. This is why we are affected by the radiations of our own sun, the stars of the zodiac, other stars and, indirectly, the moon and planets of the solar system.

An individual's astrological chart shows which light bodies can have a strong effect on the life path and we should not forget that we chose a particular star configuration to coincide with the time of our birth. (Note: For some people, stars other than the zodiac, such as Sirius, the Pleiades and the Great Bear, have a far more important role, so that care should be taken in assessing the influence of conventional astrological charts.) We can choose to align ourselves with these influences or not and the energetic effects of our choices, if any, are channelled by the etheric and communicated to the mind, emotions and body.

OUR NEED FOR THE LIGHT

If we do not have a spiritual focus, we tend to align ourselves more closely with being human, human crises, with the planetary aspects of being human and with the planet itself.

This is why our bodies, minds and emotions are today mirroring the physical pollution (earth, air, water) and abuse and destruction of planetary life. Physical, mental and/or emotional degradation in life is reflected in physical breakdown, mental and emotional suffering.

A serious consequence of too close an alignment with humanness and losing touch with the spiritual is that there is a reduction in the light that can be accommodated in the system. This is a further threat to life, to health and well-being.

Our body is doing its best to show us how, because we come from the (spiritual) light, we need this in our life. It is our main source of nourishment, yet it is one of those soul messages we only half hear. For many, the annual escape to the sun suffices!

The Source has responded to these conditions in many ways. For some time now, high frequency energies have been beamed at this planet to raise our consciousness. There are many prominent beings here, who are reminding us that we are light and we can be human. Other beings, known as *avatars* (Sanskrit, an incarnation of the Source), bring the light, show the light and infuse the consciousness of the people with the light.

Avatars, such as Sai Baba (see in Glossary), are visiting as humans, but they are embodiments of Love. They are gifting us, the Earth and the Earth family with what we need – the light. (At a world conference in India in 1968, Sai Baba declared: 'This is a human form in which every Divine entity and every divine Principle are manifest.')

ETHERIC CONSCIOUSNESS AND HEALING

Because of the close affinity between the etheric and the light, we are affected by the quantity and quality of the light that is channelled in healing. The etheric consciousness decides the destination of the light (as healing energies). Remember, etheric consciousness is soul-directed.

In our work with individuals and groups, we have observed that decisions are based on whether people need to be more human, to be more light/spiritual or to be more of both. Then, via the system of energy centres, healing is channelled to the level where it is required.

For example, one patient may need more energy for the physical body or to help them to cope with the physical circumstances being experienced. Here, the healing is helping the patient to be more human.

When the patient has over-identified with the human condition and needs to be reminded of their spiritual origins, they need to be more light-oriented. In these situations, healing often brings about dramatic changes of perspective, which may initiate major life changes in relationships, career, life path and so on. When etheric consciousness decides that the person needs to be more balanced between human and the light/spiritual, the healing manifests on the emotional and mental levels, causing changes in ways of thinking and feeling that facilitate the re-entry of light and give a spiritual perspective to experience.

If a person's experience as a human is drawing to a close, light will not be made available to the physical. Instead it is directed to the mental and/or emotional levels and will be used to help the person pass over to the next level of experience.

With practice, the healer becomes familiar with the pattern of etheric activity in individual patients so that the energetic events of the healing session can be matched with the patient's story.

What Healing Is Really For

We are convinced that, because patients are light/spiritual beings, behind the call to deal with bad backs, mental and emotional problems, and so on, healers are really being called to attend to whether a person is needing to be more human, more light, or to be a balance of both. Spiritual Healing honours the human experience of the person by holding it in the light.

This is why any form of healing that is going down the purely medical route is in danger of focusing on the human and ignoring the light being, whereas any form of health care that has a sacred perspective has this dual vision of the person as both human and light being.

In Spiritual Healing, healers have to make sure that they are not too weighted towards the human, or the light body or too mind-developed. They need to be a harmonious blend of all three. Here is a light-hearted way to assess where you are:

ACTION POINT 22 Assessing Your Balance

Developmental tool – promoting awareness of the need regularly to monitor one's activity as a spiritual being with a physical body, who experiences life on planet Earth, via mind and emotion.

This exercise may also be used as a self-healing activity. At the end of a week take a little time to work with this Action Point in your journal.

- As you review your week, how do you think you celebrated being human? Think about how you related to your body, the planet, animals and plants, food, clothes, your home, and so on.

- As you review your week, how do you think you celebrated being light? Think about your spiritual life, your love life, and other relationships at this level.

- As you review your week, how often did your conditioned mind decide how you behaved, how you felt, what you thought was 'right', how you judged yourself and others?

- As you review your week, how do you think you celebrated being both human and soul? You can decide what you think this means in terms of your own life and way of being.

- Well, where is the harmonious blend you are creating? Is there a need for adjustments anywhere?

Material about spiritual healing often refers to its purpose as being 'to restore balance and harmony'. This is not simply the restoration of balance between the systems of the body, nor a balance between the different levels of a person's being. The purpose of healing is to restore harmony between the human aspect and the light aspect of our being. In this state of balance, soul may express itself through the human in a truly creative way.

Who you are is what you offer your patients and the world. Be seriously light-hearted in your approach to this.

We can now explore soul's expression in different life situations and health conditions through the operation of the system of etheric energy centres.

8

Seven Sacred Steps

THE SEVEN SACRED STEPS IN HISTORY

In the Mithraic mysteries, souls were thought to be making a journey through seven levels of existence, pictured as a seven-stepped ladder. Later, the Gnostics, who flourished in the first three centures of the Common Era, incorporated this image into their vision of the soul journeying through seven planetary spheres. Both the ladder of Mithraism and the spheres of the Gnostics were symbols of the path into and out of incarnation. Many other ancient traditions have used the sevenfold path to describe the evolutionary path of the soul. The Seventh Heaven of the Talmud, for example, is the highest place of bliss for the returning soul.

Like the seven colours of the rainbow, seven seems to be a number of completion or perfection. It is interesting to surmise, in the light of our current knowledge, whether the sevenfold path could be the human journey through the seven main energy centres or whether this is an echo of a greater cosmic odyssey.

Information about the etheric body and its seven main energy centres passed into European culture via the civilizations of Greece and Rome. Even though it was suppressed by the fearful institutions of Catholic Christianity, the information was again conveyed to Europe through its links with the Middle Eastern, Jewish and Arab worlds. Then, in spite of the persecution and destruction of the Knights Templar (1118–1312), who came to be the guardians of this knowledge, it survived in hidden libraries and secret societies devoted to the Ageless Wisdom or classical mysteries. We see it surfacing, for example, in the work of the German mystics Jacob Boehme (1575-1624) and his pupil Johann Gichtel (1638–1710).

Today, the branch of subtle energy medicine known as chakra psychology identifies seven phases in the process of self-discovery, which are initiated by the etheric consciousness of the centres. Before we discuss the sevenfold path through the centres, we will first look at the system itself to see how the centres function individually and as a whole.

THE ACTIVITIES OF THE SEVEN MAIN CENTRES

Practice shows that the centres enable us to process our interactions with the various stages of life through which we all pass. While specific processes are going on in each centre, the system operates as a complete and interconnected whole and, through etheric consciousness, the centres are aware of all the activities in the system.

The centres may be observed as slight depressions in the luminous web-like surface of the etheric body, in which the motion of energy creates a vortex of light. Each centre is joined to a central channel, aligned with the physical spine, which is in turn connected to a network of many other channels running through the etheric. This network provides the basis of the meridian system known to those practising acupuncture, Shiatsu and traditional Chinese Medicine.

During the operation of a centre, the vortex of light moves out from the surface of the etheric body to project into the energy field. It now appears as a bell-shaped or funnel-shaped structure connected at its narrower end to the central channel. Just like the main body of the etheric, the structure is formed by a grid-like pattern of light. Its bell-like shape facilitates the gathering or emission of energies.

The etheric acts as the communication vehicle for soul, enabling the passage of energies from soul to the physical and from the physical back to the soul. Thus, the centres act as a distribution system for all the energies, including the emotional and mental, that are generated during a person's life experience.

Another of the functions of the centres is to identify subtle energies and, if possible, to process them. Very often a person is not ready to deal with a certain situation, such as a bereavement, so that etheric consciousness directs these energies to be stored for processing later.

However, the system is designed to alert us to the presence of stored, unprocessed material. Through what we have discussed already, it can be understood that the alarm signal could take the form of mental or emotional distress or physical ill health.

There is more about the movement of subtle energies into the body in Chapter 10, The Travelling Structure.

THE ENERGIES OF LIFE

Last, but not least, the centres are responsible for conveying the life force (*prana* in Sanskrit, *ki* in Japanese, *qi* in Chinese) to the physical where it interacts with every cell in the body, infusing them with that animation we call 'life'.

Two vitality energies permeate the physical and other levels, via the sacral and solar plexus centres. The vitality energy of the sacral is essential to creativity, the generation of joy and the creative expression of our sexuality. The release of these energies depends to some extent on this centre's contact with the spiritual forces of the soul.

The vitality energy of the solar plexus is essential to our sense of being a whole person and to the active strength of the will. Again, the release of these energies depends to an extent on the contact of soul energy with this centre. When these contacts are not made, the force of the centres tends to be directed on behalf of the personality's needs and desires alone.

THE SEVEN CENTRES AND THE CENTRES OF THE HANDS AND FEET

There are some 360 light centres in the etheric body, most of which have specific links with the functioning of the physical. Your awareness of these links will grow with experience.

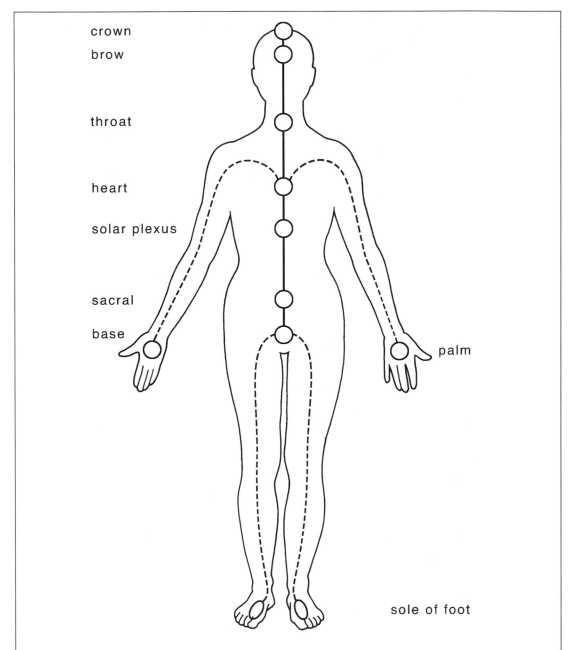

crown

brow

throat

heart

solar plexus

sacral

base

palm

sole of foot

Figure 20. The principal energy centres used in healing – showing links between palm and heart, sole and base.

Our work over 15 years has shown us that the seven main energy centres, their function and disfunction, are those most directly related to our life journey, to our health and well-being, and are the centres most directly concerned with healing. For this reason, it is important to fully understand the function of the seven main centres and the four related centres in the feet and hands.

First, we will look at the centres of the hands and feet and their important links with the main system. The centres in the soles of the feet absorb energies from the core of the Earth and the surface layer of the planet on which life depends. This is why it is good to go barefoot on the Earth when you can. These centres link the polarity of the planetary energies with the two etheric polarity channels. They act as grounding or earthing points, as does the base centre, for incoming subtle energies.

In the subtle energy science of Qi Gong (see Glossary), the *yongquan* point on the sole of the foot is connected to the kidneys and is also used in cases of hypertension. This meridian point is in the same place as the sole-of-the-foot centre and its function gives a clue to the link between the centres of the feet and the base (since the energies of the base centre enter the physical body via the adrenal glands).

ACTION POINT 23 Sensing the Energies of the Planet

Developmental tool – promoting awareness of and sensitivity to the subtle energy systems of the planet.

This exercise may also be used as a self-healing technique to absorb basic Earth energies.

- Stand on the ground with bare feet in a relaxed posture. Use the breath to bring balance to the body.

- Put your mind in the soles of your feet. Be aware of your contact with the ground, with the body of Mother Earth, with the grass, the soil, sand or whatever is under your feet. Close your eyes and see if you sense an energetic transaction via the soles of your feet.

- Still with your focus in the feet, use the in-breath to aid your awareness of the passage of energy from your feet, up your legs to the centre at the base of your spine. Inhale a few times with this intention.

- Make a note of your discoveries. Repeat the exercise in different locations and at different times of the day and night. Again, what did you discover?

The centres of the hand connect the two polarity channels with the polarity of the energy field. This does not affect the flow of energy via either hand in healing.

In Qi Gong, the *laogong* point on the palm of the hand is related to the heart, blood circulation and to the release of negative *qi* (heavy energy). This clue tells us about the link between the centres of the palms and the heart, the important link that allows us to give healing with the hands. Let's see if you can sense this important energy circuit.

ACTION POINT 24 Sensing Energy with the Palm Centres

Developmental tool – promoting awareness of subtle energy exchange, and the giving and receiving capacities of palmar energetic structures.

This exercise may also be used as a self-healing technique, encouraging openness and the ability to give and receive love.

The exercise is in two parts. The first part focuses on drawing in energy, the second on giving it out.

- Stand or sit in a relaxed posture, with the legs uncrossed. Hold your palms out in front of you. Relax your elbows, the back of the neck and the shoulders. Close your eyes if this helps concentration.

- Focus your attention on the palm centres. As you inhale, sense that you can draw energy in through the palm centres. Breathe out gently, through the palms. What are your sensations with both parts of the breath?

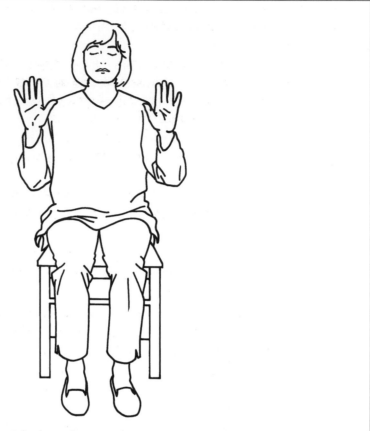

Figure 21. Sensing energy with the palms.

- Now visualize the energetic link between your palms and your heart centre. Breathe in and sense energy moving up your arms, across the shoulders, to converge in the centre of your chest, in the heart centre.

- Lower your arms and relax for a few moments.

- Raise your arms again with your hands held in front of you as before. In this second part of the exercise, you are going to send energy from the heart to the palms.

- Close the eyes if this helps concentration. Focus on the heart centre and relax. Breathe into the heart centre. As you exhale, visualize energy moving from the heart centre, out to the shoulders, down the arms, to the centre in each palm, and out. What do you sense this time?

● Compare notes about absorbing and transmitting energy through the palm and heart centres.

The experiences you have gained with the last two Action Points should reinforce your understanding of their role in healing. The sole centres, through their contact with the planet, keep us grounded energetically. This is important for our efficient functioning as a channeller of the light and for the channelling of the light to the patient. If the patient has left the physical body during the healing session (a common occurrence), their attention is drawn to the body, the feet and to their connection with the ground.

Through the centres in the hands, we transmit the light (healing energy) and we absorb energetic information. During this activity, especially during the healing scans, the palm centres act like a kind of subtle eye. If we are soul-centred, we are heart-centred and we can depend on the hands, through their link with the heart, to carry out the healing just as it is required by soul.

So we are in touch with the Earth with our feet and we are in touch with soul through our hands. These four centres provide us with an opportunity to celebrate our love for the Earth (perhaps through dance and movement) and our love for the Earth family (perhaps through using the hands to heal, comfort, prepare food, make ceremony and make music).

MOVEMENT OF THE ENERGIES

Energies from the planet (physical level), the base, sacral and solar plexus centres move up the system via the central channel. The vibrations of the centres become relatively faster from the base to the crown so that incoming energies are modified/processed before they can flow on up the system.

Energies from the soul/spiritual (light level) move down through the crown, brow and throat centres, via the central channel. Again, they are modified/processed before they can flow on down through the system.

The heart centre is the mid-point of these two flows of energy and is effectively the balancing agent of the whole subtle energy system.

The flow of energies from the realms of the Earth and the spirit proclaim the essential identity of us humans – we are light beings expressing ourselves through the sacred human. It is the job of the etheric centres to help us develop and maintain a harmonious balance of these two aspects of soul – the light and the human. This harmony is exhibited in the down-to-earth person who radiates light, love and peace into the world. Do you know someone like this?

Now let's make sure you can locate the seven main centres by sensing them with the hands. As well as with groups of healing trainees, we have used Action Points 25 and 26 (below) with doctors, nurses, psychologists and psychotherapists. Every group has been amazed how easy it was to sense the energy centres.

ACTION POINT 25 Sensing the Location of the Seven Centres – Patient on the Healing Couch

Developmental tool – increasing sensitivity to and awareness of the principle structures within the subtle energy system, using the palms.

- Have your partner remove their shoes and lie on the healing couch on their back. They should relax with their hands at their sides and breathe normally. Stand next to their head, ready to sense the crown centre.

- Raise your hands up above the region of your partner's crown centre with the arms fully extended. Your palms should be about 20 to 30cm apart.

- Slowly lower your arms, allowing your palms to move down towards the crown centre. Bear in mind that, although the centre may be sensed at an etheric level (some 5 to 10cm from the body), there may be a need for energy at the mental or emotional level. Therefore, feel carefully for a 'resistance' of energy against your palms. As soon as you feel this resistance (like a slight pressure), keep the hands at this spot.

- This is the location of the crown centre. Notice where its energies extend to in the field.

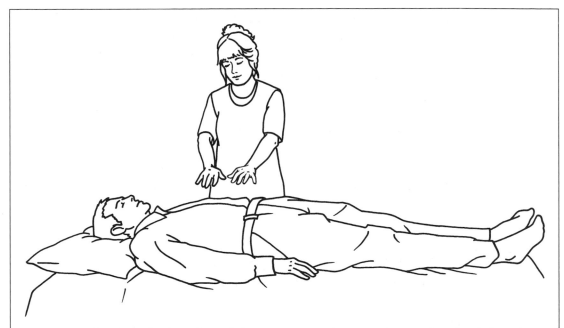

Figure 22. Sensing the location of the centres, patient on the couch – both hands are locating the solar plexus centre.

- Now raise your arms and move both hands to a position over the brow centre. Again, lower your arms until you feel a pressure against your palms from your partner's brow. This is its location.

- Raise your arms and move your hands above the throat. Repeat the procedure over the heart, solar plexus, sacral and base centres to locate them. At the base centre, move your hands slowly away from your partner's body.

- Allow your partner to sit up on the couch. Discuss your findings. What was your partner aware of during your sensing?

- Now take the place of your partner and allow them to locate your seven centres. Discuss and compare your findings.

Though a healing couch is generally preferable, sometimes you will need to work on a chair. This is the case when the patient cannot lie down in comfort, for example. When using a chair, the same procedures as above are followed, but notice the change in the position of the hands.

> **ACTION POINT 26 Sensing the Location of the Centres – Patient on the Healing Chair**

Developmental tool – increasing sensitivity to and awareness of the principle structures within the subtle energy system, using the palms.

- Your partner should be seated with their legs and arms uncrossed, and the hands resting on the thighs. They should relax and breathe normally.

- Stand behind your partner and raise your hands up above the partner's crown centre with the arms fully extended. Your palms should be about 20 to 30cm apart.

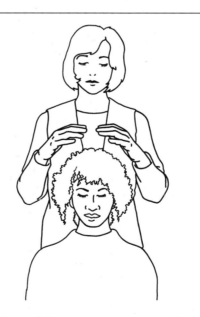

Figure 23. Sensing the location of the crown centre, patient on the chair.

- Slowly lower your arms, allowing your palms to move down towards the crown centre until you sense a pressure against the palms. Stop at this point. Notice where the crown energies extend to in the energy field.

- Step to one side of your partner while you move your hands to either side of the brow centre with your arms extended. Slowly bring them in towards the brow until you feel the pressure of energy against your palms. Stop at this point and notice where the brow energies extend to in the field.

- Move to the throat. Again, extend your arms away from the throat and slowly bring them together to locate the energies of the centre.

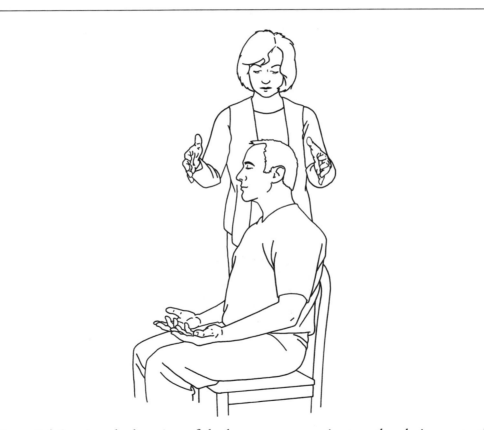

Figure 24. Sensing the location of the brow centre, patient on the chair – note the position to sense both energy projections of the centre.

- Use the same procedure with the heart, solar plexus and sacral centres. You may find you need to kneel on the ground or to use a chair to sit on so that you are comfortable while working with the lower centres. It is important to relax to be fully sensitive.

- The curvature of the body when sitting means that the base centre is sensed with the hands at an angle of about 45 degrees. Proceed in the same way as before.

- What was your partner aware of during your sensing?

- Change over and compare notes with your partner.

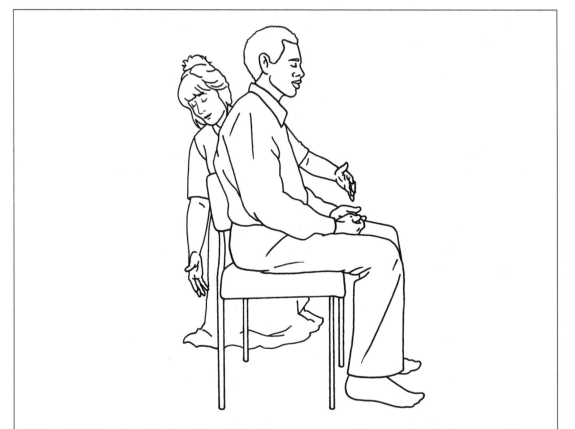

Figure 25. Sensing the location of the base centre, patient on the chair – note the 45 degree angle of the energy projections.

You will notice that it was not necessary to hold the hands on both sides of the centres when working with the couch. In fact, the centres may be sensed in all directions, as if they were spherical. It is your intention that is important.

Working Intuitively With The Centres

Intuitive assessment of the centre scans provides an energetic diagnosis, which must then be matched to the patient's story and the pattern of the healing. Your intuitive work with the centres and etheric consciousness is the outcome of the presenting condition and its cause, the patient's way of seeing it and the soul's directions on what needs to be done. Ian's story provides us with a number of learning points.

Called to a home visit, I found Ian's limp body lying in his bed. The healing scans reflected the physical picture. There was hardly sufficient life force to maintain Ian's system. The heart and base chakras were closed. The solar plexus centre was drained and the brow abnormally extended. The sacral and throat centres were barely detectable. The crown was functioning but damaged. The energy circuits were seriously under-functioning.

Ian was very ill. He had suffered from ME (Chronic Fatigue Syndrome) for five years. He had been making good progress, but a relapse six months before had resulted in his present poor state. He wondered if healing could help.

The condition ME is perhaps the most dramatic subtle energy pattern for a healer to meet since it mimics death – the gradual withdrawal of the life force from the physical body. There is no part of the human system that is not affected. In severe cases the ME patient experiences severe mental and emotional disturbance, with depression and interrupted thinking processes, in addition to the distress of physical immobility.

Over a ten-year period of working with many patients with ME, a clear pattern has emerged:

- The base and heart chakras are always affected – without exception.

- The condition mimics the energy pattern associated with human death.
- There is always an element of loss in the patient's story, although it may take some considerable time for this to make itself known. The unresolved issue around the loss is the trigger for the emotional and mental systems to break down. Family and friends are usually unaware of the nature of the loss. It may go back many years in the patient's life.
- ME patients are either unable to generate sufficient life force to maintain the system or a part of the system or they are able to generate life force but unable to retain it for the well-being of the system.
- The energy circuits are interrupted and in extreme cases are barely functioning.
- The healing scans will indicate to the intuitive healer where the healing needs to begin – energy centre or skeletal energy circuit or auric zone.

Ian was 32, a successful businessman, married with a young daughter. The onset of ME had been a gradual process.

From the first session, in six months Ian moved from barely registering my presence, to sitting up and looking forward to my visits, to welcoming me at the front door.

He continued his weekly healing sessions at the clinic. There he occasionally reviewed how successful he was at his job and how he was looking forward to doing some work from home before returning to the office. Whenever he spoke in this way his energy system would react – effectively limiting the energy available to his system.

Despite this, his sacral centre would open fully, in response to my hands, calling for more and more energy. What was happening? I felt that I knew quite a lot about Ian's story by now, but realized at no time had he mentioned anything to do with creativity. Could this be a clue to his condition? Ian could experience the change in healing energy when his sacral centre was reacting.

'What does the sacral centre do?' he asked. 'It processes the energy of sexuality, how you celebrate being male. It's the place of your inner child and, oh yes, creativity,' I replied. There was that word – creativity! Ian's eyes lit up and then he started to cry. Soon he was sobbing. Between the sobs emerged the story of a young man who had wanted to study art and become an artist. His family had disapproved and insisted that he study economics and business.

This was a breakthrough, but Ian despaired, 'It's all too late, too late. My wife married a businessman not an artist. I'll lose my wife and family if I go down that track!'

Despite his protestations, in his healing sleeps during subsequent sessions he was reminded of how creative he was. He would see himself painting and he could smell the paint. He still maintained that it was all too late, but he would agree to some homework where he would try and record one or two of the paintings he saw himself doing – just to keep me happy and, yes, he would bring them in.

Although Ian despaired of it being too late, his health was suggesting otherwise. As Ian picked up his brushes his health continued to improve. I felt privileged to witness the birth of a very talented artist.

On a wall in the clinic hangs the painting of a scene in Italy where Ian and his family now live, signed by all of them. Ian says he hopes it will be an inspiration to others.

Pondering over Ian's story, I wondered at his soul assuming control and withdrawing energy from a way of life that was completely incompatible so that it could be reinvested in a new way of being.

THE CHALLENGE OF THE SEVEN SACRED STEPS

When we consider the sevenfold journey through the centres, we begin to see what an adventure life is and how finding the harmony mentioned above is no mean achievement. For most of us, making the trip from base to crown alone will merit a gold medal. Bearing in mind all the energetic movements and flows described so far, let us look at the challenges presented by the Seven Sacred Steps.

The base centre – the first Sacred Step

Soul rejoices in the Earth and has embedded itself deep in physical experience, so the first Sacred Step is the base centre, opposite the base of the spine. This centre processes all issues of how we relate to physicality. Do we like being here? Do we honour the Earth and the Earth family? Do we like our bodies and do we honour them? Do we realize that our sensual awareness is for soul's delight and not a problem for the personality? These are some of the questions you have to answer as truthfully as possible. Remember, you are the only listener and you are the only judge. Can you stop being the judge and just be loving with yourself?

We are made from the Earth and this is our human home for the time being. Do we feel safe and secure, or is our survival threatened in some way? This question affects us when we are still in the womb and for many it continues to be the most important question of base centre experience.

When this centre is calling for energy, a patient may be dealing with one or more of the issues we have mentioned. Finally, there is a dormant energy stored in the base, which can be likened to a coiled spring or an egg in its shell (known in Sanskrit as *kundalini*, from *kundal*, 'coil' and its feminine ending *ini*). This is the energy of spiritual awakening that reminds us of our true origins. As we bring our centres into balance and harmony through properly processing all of life's energetic material, we clear the central channel (like clearing the 'hollow bone' or healing channel). Once the channel is clear the base centre, representing our physical being, can hear the call of the soul. The dormant energy responds by breaking out of its 'shell' and moving up the central channel, gathering power and speed as it progresses. When this highly potent energy reaches the crown it is like the meeting of two long-lost lovers – soul meets soul, light meets light.

There are systems of exercises, such as those of kundalini yoga, which speed up the movement of energy through the centres. But if the kundalini is forced up the central channel before it is clear enough, the impact of the energy on the centres may cause mental and/or psychological pain. For this reason these systems should only be practised under the guidance of reliable and experienced teachers. Rest assured that when your system is ready you will know intuitively and everything will happen quite naturally at the right time. There is no need to rush things.

When in a state of balance, the light of the base centre vibrates as the colour red.

The sacral centre – the second Sacred Step

From the moment that we feel safe and secure, we take the second Sacred Step into the sacral centre, which is opposite the sacral bones of the spine, just below the navel. The balanced centre vibrates with an orange light.

Here we process all the issues connected with our creativity, sexuality and experiences of joy. Creativity is the second sphere of experience and urges us to be artists of life. You may not be a painter or a musician, but bringing a child into the world is a supreme act of creation. If this has not been part of your life, you prepare food, dress yourself and have a living and work space to look after. There are a hundred-and-one ways to be creative in life.

The second challenge of this centre is how we relate to and express our sexuality. It is always part of us, whether we express it or not. The urge to have sex is not simply the urge to procreate, rather it is the signal to experience Oneness. When all the centres are engaged in sex, not just the base and sacral, orgasm is experienced as the rise of the life force up the central channel to the brow centre. The ecstasy of orgasm tells us about the ecstasy of Oneness. The goal is not to restrict ourselves to the sexual form alone.

In the sacral centre, we honour the inner child. We learn to play and in playing we release the energy of joy that may be felt as a powerful emotion. Joy acts as a yardstick against which we compare the other emotions we feel. 'Does it give you joy?' can be an important question in assessing how you really feel about something. Children, especially, demonstrate the release of joy energy when they giggle. The 'giggle factor' is the clue to joyfulness.

All these energies move to the throat centre to be expressed and there is a special link between these two centres.

The solar plexus centre – the third Sacred Step

Our sense of personal self and personal power is generated in this centre, situated just below the diaphragm and above the navel. The balanced solar plexus centre vibrates with a golden yellow light.

The third Sacred Step challenges us to see how far life experience has empowered us or disempowered us, and how we react to people and situations in terms of our sense of self. This sense of self has been created by our mind as we have grown, developed, experienced life and reacted to the behaviour of others.

This centre processes all issues connected with the mind and our thoughts, confronting us with our conditioned mind patterns. It has been designed to record and remember and this is what it does. But we find that not all of our mind's conditioning is conducive to our well-being.

Mind's impact with physical life generates feelings and emotions and this centre also deals with the effects of all our emotional issues.

We can appreciate that the three steps we have taken so far are very much to do with our humanness. The next step will make us look back at these three to see if we have processed their energies and to see if we have been able to act with love or otherwise.

The heart centre – the fourth Sacred Step

Situated midway between the base and the crown, the fourth Sacred Step is found in the centre of the chest. This is considered the place of the soul and it is where soul 'speaks' to us. To express the light of the soul as love is the challenge of the heart centre, which deals with all issues of love and lovelessness in our life. The balanced centre vibrates with a green light, the colour of balance.

It can be seen that when the hands are held by the sides of the body they are in line with the base centre. This relationship between the heart and the base centre is frequently demonstrated through the hands. We have worked with patients where the eczema on the hands had a direct relationship with issues of love, lovelessness and survival.

We are living at a time when the balance point of the centres is the crisis point in human affairs. Love has been your greatest challenge so far and will continue to be so. Do you love yourself and do you love yourself as the Source? Do you love others (because of Oneness) and can you love without judging? Is 'love and light' a mere fashionable phrase or a radiation from you into the world? These are some of the questions by which the heart centre asks you how conditional or unconditional your love really is. Your heart knows and it cannot be fooled!

The heart centre balances the energies of spirit moving down the system and the energies of physical life moving up. In all cases the heart is monitoring how much the personality is involved, how much the soul is involved and the balance between them.

The challenge for us at this time of crisis is whether we will move from a fear-based way of being (which will keep us in the solar plexus centre, in the grip of mind) to a love-based way of being (which will need us to be heart-centred). We have had thousands of years of knowing what fear would do in a given situation. Now we need to ask: 'What would love do?'.

Love will give an answer to any problem, on any occasion. For when the heart is asked it is soul that replies and shows us the way through to the light. Soul's answer makes everybody happy and everyone wins.

The throat centre – the fifth Sacred Step

Do not be surprised if you find yourself lingering for some time on step four. But we have to express who we are and the throat calls.

The fifth Sacred Step is located, as its name implies, in the throat. The challenge here is to be authentic. The throat centre processes all issues of expression and communication, and all the different ways that we use to express ourselves and communicate with others. The balanced centre vibrates with a sky blue light.

The throat asks, 'Do you express who you really are or only part of yourself or a distorted aspect of yourself? Do you treasure the truth or is the lie OK?' The problem with the lie is that it is saying, 'I'm not OK, you are not OK, they are not OK, life is not OK and soul is not OK.'

Lies accumulate energies like themselves so that whole areas of our being and our life become weighed down with the heavy energy of falsehood and negativity. They have no power to do any good, even though this may have been our motive in lying.

In the other centres it may take time before we are aware of a block in the system, but if we suppress the *expression* of any of the subtle energies, we feel a pain or block in the throat straight away.

The throat centre is an expression of the light aspect, so it is very much concerned with truth and authenticity. Here we learn to trust soul, to trust the soul in others and in life.

The brow centre – the sixth Sacred Step

As we take the sixth Sacred Step to the brow centre, our trust in soul is challenged straight away. Here, in the centre of the forehead, just above the brows, we receive information from our psychic awareness (the 'sixth sense') and our intuitive awareness (the 'seventh sense'). *Psychic awareness* enables us to be aware of subtle energetic phenomena, such as the light of the aura for example, which are external to us. On the other hand, *intuitive awareness* enables us to be aware of the messages of soul and information from the spiritual levels, which are energies that are internal to us. The brow centre also receives and processes subtle energetic information from the etheric consciousness. The balanced centre vibrates to a deep royal blue or indigo light.

Our problem with all of the inputs to the brow is that once they are conveyed to the brain for interpretation, the mind acts as uninvited consultant, only able to compare information received with what it already knows. If mind cannot match the information with our perceived life experience, it tends to put it in the reject tray.

When intuition is properly heard, uncontaminated by mind, it will be seen to be 'right'. You can probably recall times when you had a hunch, then you thought about it and it did not seem such a good idea after all, so you did not act on it. Later you discovered that your hunch was right, if only you had followed it. This is how mind messes with intuition, soul knowledge.

The brow centre is the place where truth is tested. It is also the place where all energies destined for the crown are monitored to see if they have been fully processsed. If not, they are sent back to where they originated.

We all have lots of fun and games with the brow centre. It has been called the Third Eye since ancient times because it seemed to be another way of seeing beyond the ordinary or the appearance of things. This is exactly what it can do, in terms of our psychic and intuitive awareness. For healers the brow is the intuitive link with soul and the soul of the patient.

The crown centre – the seventh Sacred Step

The crown centre is our link with the Source and the Light, and the seventh Sacred Step may seem daunting. On the crown of the head, this centre deals with all issues of our spirituality. It is the first centre representing our light aspect and the challenge is to acknowledge this and allow it to have full expression in our life. The balanced centre vibrates with a violet or purple light.

The crown has a special link with the base and this tells us that it is not a question of our being either spiritual or human, but of owning up to being an embodiment of the light. And so, as we take this seventh step, we find we have discovered the human rainbow or spectrum of light inside ourselves. It is as if we have shown ourselves that our life is actually a complete whole and that there is no issue or experience that does not have a valid place in our story.

The lower three centres, via the mind, exert a pressure on the personality to engage in humanness as if that was all there is. The upper three centres of the crown, brow and throat, via our intuition and feelings, exert a pressure on the personality to recall our light origins.

The heart shows us that we will only ever be half what we could be until we make the leap of faith and trust in our reality as soul. Through its processing of love issues, the heart centre also shows us that love is the key to a harmonious balance of both aspects of our being. This is the soul message that is sent to us by the crown and heart centres.

THE LINKS BETWEEN THE CENTRES

There is no division between the lower three and the upper three centres. The whole system is an essential unity of the human and the light aspects of the soul. This is reflected in the five special energetic links between the centres. During the healing scans, as well as working with each centre, the healer also works to reinforce and heal the five links (see Chapter 14, The Sacred Meeting):

- **Base-Heart** This link affirms the place of the body within the soul. It is a link of love with the body and the planet. This link is weakened through conditions such as the loss of a loved one, where the person feels their own survival or place in the world is now threatened. It can also be weakened through failure to love one's own body.
- **Sacral-Throat** This link facilitates the expression of all creativity. When issues in either centre dominate, they may block the flow of energy through this link.
- **Solar Plexus-Brow** This link allows soul knowledge from the brow to be checked out by mind and for mental material to be checked out by intuition. Where mind or emotions become dominant, the voice of intuition is either not heard or not heeded.
- **Heart-Crown** This link affirms the place of soul in the heart. Its perma-

nent link to the source of love supports the balancing function of the heart. Our reaction to life experiences may block the flow of unconditional love.

- **Base-Crown** This affirms the link between the Source and the physical, the link of Oneness. It unites our spirituality with our physical life. Our reaction to life experiences may block the flow of spiritual nourishment into our life.

Checking centre energies and centre links

Patsy's story, below, shows the importance of understanding the links between the centres and how they impact on the body. Here, Patsy's body sends a signal with clues about the cause of her ill health.

> Patsy was 29 and losing her hearing. Medical investigation had found no reason for the condition. Her voice would disappear for weeks at a time. In desperation Patsy turned to healing.
>
> During the healing scans a pearlescent luminous energy was present in and around the sacral energy centre. This is normally associated with pregnancy and yet Patsy had made no reference to a pregnancy in the telling of her story. After the healing I asked Patsy if she had ever been pregnant. Patsy broke down in tears. Yes, she had been pregnant but her boyfriend insisted that she had an abortion. She never told any of her friends or family. Following the abortion her boyfriend left her. Patsy's choking sobs filled the room.
>
> Her sacral centre still bore the energetic scars of the abortion and the trace energy of the unborn child. The sacral centre was shut down and the link centre, the throat chakra, was badly affected by having to cope with the energetic function of the two chakras. This impacted on Patsy's hearing and voice.
>
> Over the weeks healing helped Patsy to heal the grief and guilt she felt over the abortion. As the healing progressed the luminescent energy disappeared and the sacral and throat centres were restored. Her hearing returned and she had no further problems with her voice.

Did you notice the sacral-throat energy link? Practice shows that, by the time disharmony is manifesting on the physical, it has already affected the related centre and at least one other. So you should always check the energies of those centres above and below the related centre, as well as that to which it is linked. It was this procedure that brought about the total healing in Patsy's case.

SEVEN LEVELS OF CONSCIOUSNESS

Soul prepared the path and life arranges experiences for us to journey towards and through the seven Sacred Steps or phases of being human. Each step is like an initiation, rather like the initiatory aspect of the healing session. Our encounter with the centres does not take place in such an orderly sequence, but our processing of their energies imposes its own progression. This is because the centres are levels of consciousness and therefore levels of healing. For all of us, the invitation of the seven Sacred Steps is to raise our energy to the highest level possible in every moment. This finds its fullest expression when we can consciously engage all seven centres in what we are doing.

Following the awakening of all the seven centres, we are able to give light out to the world. This is represented in images of the Buddha by the everted crown centre (often shown as a topknot of hair) and in Christian and Hindu images by a halo of light around the head.

Many indigenous societies recognized this phenomenon in light-filled chiefs, teachers, medicine people and tribal leaders, of both sexes, by awarding them headdresses of feathers. Since large birds are considered to be the messengers of the Source (Great Spirit), the feathered bonnet of the Native American Indians, for example, has considerable significance. In many world cultures, including western cultures, the golden crown became the enduring symbol of the enlightened leader/ruler.

The healer can help the patient to reclaim those etheric centres of life that have been closed off, avoided or only half engaged with. Much of the unprocessed energy released will have been stored at the mental or emotional level of the energy field. It is to these aspects of being human that we turn next.

9

Sacred Mind –
Sacred Feeling

SOUL'S INSTRUMENTS

Life here is for soul's purpose and soul has a range of instruments that allow it to totally engage in the physical and to endow it with sacred life. We have seen how the etheric body was created to be soul's vehicle for communication. Now we look at how mind and emotion enable us to transform soul's message into the activities of the physical body.

Mind is the mechanism whereby the will of soul can be expressed. This means that we can use our mind to create and to make things happen. It helps us to organize what needs to be done through its three facets of thought, intellect (which allows us to choose) and will (which is the power behind the mind's choice).

Emotions and feelings are the soul language that enables us to interpret the 'rightness' (for us) of what is happening. We use emotions to monitor our journey of experience – to feel how it is going and how in keeping we are with our own sacred purpose.

If we recall the route of the soul message (see Figure 19 in Chapter 7), soul indicates its desire through its call or message, the sacred language of soul. The message is communicated to us via the centres of the etheric body. First, mind's function is to check the message and to choose (from the alternatives in its databank of previous experience) what to do and how to do it. Next, the function of emotion is to feel the substance of the soul message and what does or does not feel right about mind's choice of what to do. Finally, the function of the body is to put the mind's choice into action. Emotion then registers how it feels for the body to be acting in this way.

Before we look at how the implementation of soul's message is crucial to our health and well-being, we will sum up the function of each of the aspects of what makes us human.

We are soul, the instrument of the Source. This is our true self. Life is the creation of soul:

- **The etheric** (an instrument of soul) communicates all that is happening to all levels.
- **Mind** (an instrument of soul) makes choices based on what it knows and its conditioned programmes.
- **Emotion** (an instrument of soul) is a signalling system that monitors the relationship between soul and mind and tells us who is in control. Feelings tell us if any experience is good for us or not.
- **Body** (an instrument of soul) actively carries out soul's message, as it has been interpreted and conveyed by mind.
- **Personality/ego** (an instrument of soul) is the sum total of all the characteristics of the physical, emotional and mental aspects by which an individual is recognized as unique. Soul's mission is to express itself through the personality.

Where the energy field is a complete record of a person's experiences, the personality is the demonstration vehicle for those experiences.

All these aspects are linked, at a subtle level, by the energy centres, to form the total subtle energy system.

ALIGNMENT AND NON-ALIGNMENT WITH THE SOUL MESSAGE

When soul is able to create in harmony with the personality, we experience the bliss of Oneness, moments of total and deep awareness. Such moments of feeling tell us that soul's choice (not mind's choice) is being carried out.

This is ideally what would happen, but, as we saw in Ian's story in Chapter

8, for example, this is rarely the case because of our mental and/or emotional reactions to what has happened in our life, especially as children and young people. Our mental and emotional conditioning mean that, for most of us, soul's message does not get through intact and sometimes does not get through at all.

The patient's story and expressions of thought and feeling indicate alignment or non-alignment with soul. These alignments find expression as our health and well-being. This is why the task of healing is to work with the alignment of the patient with their soul mission, whether the patient is conscious of this actuality or not, whatever the condition they are presenting.

In Ian's story, his life was seriously out of alignment with his soul's desire to be creative. His soul sent a message to let him know about the misalignment. The message went first to mind. It showed Ian, by its ways of thinking, that all was not well. But mind tends to think it is all that is, that the soul does not exist and that its job is to tell the body what to do. So the message was passed to the emotional level, which showed Ian through his distress that all was not well. Still he did not recognize soul's message, which then was passed to the body. Ian's body tried to convey the urgency of soul's message through the seriousness of his condition. The lines of communication were almost blocked.

Mental Conditioning Interferes With Soul's Message

The etheric communication system enables this process to ricochet back to emotions and mind to give them further information. When the body gets sick, mind thinks that things are not as they should be and emotions tell us that something does not feel right. Mind is the first to think it can fix it and may urge us to take a pill, or some course of action. When they do not work we are impressed to try a more powerful pill, and so on. If we cannot seem to help ourselves, mind urges us to go and see someone, so we look for an answer outside of self. When we visit the doctor or therapist for help it will be rare if they say, 'Ah, there could be a soul issue here.'

So we get very little help to recognize the signals that we are out of alignment with our soul's message. Things have got to this point because we no longer know how to listen to ourselves.

But even if we do know, the listening process is often thwarted at the start by the conditioning of our minds. This is possible because mind can be trained. This is of great value unless the training or conditioning it receives is such that it acts against our best interest and distorts soul's message.

This is why personal transformation needs to be part of our spirituality. Therapy shows us how our mindsets interfere with soul's message. When we know this we are empowered to make the necessary changes to choose ways of thinking and behaving. Spiritual Healing is the perfect accompaniment to all therapies because, with its transpersonal/spiritual base, it holds the possibility of soul relationship at its core.

Ian's story describes someone whose mental conditioning prevented his soul message from getting through so that soul drew his attention to this by means of a chronic bodily condition. Healing was able to reopen the lines of communication before it was too late. Where a person has totally blocked communication and does not heed the messages of mind, body or emotions, soul may decide to leave the body. After all, it has eternity in which to express itself. In this case the healer's role is to help the patient to do this.

MIND FINDS WAYS TO BLOCK THE MESSAGE OF THE EMOTIONS

As we will see in Carol's case, below, soul's message was heard at the mental and emotional levels, and at this point Carol sought healing. Carol's story illustrates how her mind became trained so that the call of soul became distorted. Her emotions told her that what she was experiencing was definitely not good for her, but her conditioned mind found ways to block her emotional response.

Carol's journey had taken her into a series of abusive relationships, which had begun in childhood with a violent, alcoholic father. Carol and her mother had suffered considerable physical violence, and mental and emotional abuse.

As Carol told her story, detailing some of her experiences with her father, she appeared to be growing smaller in the chair and her voice became childlike in expression and sound. The child self of Carol needed to be heard.

She held herself tightly in the chair as if attempting to take up less and less space. Her breathing was also affected. With shoulders hunched and arms pinned to her sides, Carol was taking such shallow breaths that she could hardly finish a sentence.

She continued her story. 'I have to have some help to leave this marriage. If I don't I won't survive.' Her phrase hung in the air between us as we both absorbed the seriousness of her situation.

Carol said that she could see a pattern in her life of moving from one disastrous relationship to another. She wanted healing to help her grow strong and end this pattern. As she spoke, her voice changed and the adult was present once again.

The healing showed Carol that early in her life she had been the victim of a very cruel parent. As she grew up a way of thinking had grown with her. She had developed a mindset that influenced the way she felt about herself, her life and relationships, and affected the way she operated emotionally. The mindset told her that women make men angry and that was why they had to be beaten; that men were more important than women who should do what men say and what they want; that being hurt physically, mentally and emotionally was part of being a woman. 'This is what my life has been about,' she said. 'My mother's life was the same.'

Initially, whenever the healing was directed to the mental and emotional zones in Carol's aura, she would revert to her childhood state and the child would find a way of releasing the tears she had had to suppress for fear of being beaten again. The energetic material of Carol's thinking and feeling during her experiences of being abused was stored within these zones.

Healing showed that the energy of the victim needed to be released to help Carol break this pattern of behaviour. Then her aura would no longer send the subtle energetic message to a potential abuser that she was a target for further abuse.

Carol's changing voice and the material released during healing sessions showed how she was moving through her healing process. She left her marriage and in the course of 18 months Carol learned to love her body and herself. Her way of thinking about herself and her relationships changed. Her confidence and self-esteem grew.

She later wrote saying that she had joined the local college and was studying counselling.

Carol learned that her soul spoke to her in feelings, that she could listen to her feelings, follow them and honour them. She realized that if she ever needed to know what was right or true for her about something, she could go by how she felt.

How Mind Copes With Negative Experience

Mind is a reservoir of information about all our experiences. Its perception of these experiences depends on the presence or absence of love. From its perceptions it develops mindsets – ways of interpreting the world – that are established very early in life.

Sometimes healing involves helping the patient to change a mindset, so that they can open up to love, or healing the patient's experiences of lovelessness, as in Carol's case. All these heart-based healings create ways through for soul's message.

When soul sends a message to us, it encapsulates a total picture of our true reality, which is love. If this conflicts with our life experience (as when we are unloved, put down, not validated, for example, or when lovelessness takes the form of abuse at some level, as it did with Carol), the mind has to find ways to cope with the discrepency. Ways of thinking, feeling and behaving are developed accordingly.

From a place of pain the world appears frightening and cruel. Defensiveness and aggression develop and lovelessness becomes manifested in many forms.

You will recall that when Ian was quite young, he received a soul impulse to be an artist. His life experience was that this was not approved of and would not be possible. His way of coping was to become the conformist who could act out the role of the businessman and good family provider. He thought the world would not support his being an artist, but eventually his soul got its message through via the condition of ME. Through healing Ian was able to see how he had been living a false message and to renew his link with his real self and his soul's mission.

Mind, Emotions And Spiritual Growth

Soul grows and develops through all of our life experiences. Spiritual Healing understands spiritual development, from the personality point of view, as finding ways to open the channels for soul's messages so that they can be acted out in the life of the body. The purpose of personal transformation is to achieve that harmony between body, emotions, mind and soul/spirit where the message is not changed, distorted or thwarted. This state of harmony feels wonderful because we are feeling what it is like to be who we truly are.

Our emotional response to situations tells us how far we have progressed in achieving harmony. We have seen that the conditioned mind (and just living our lives always involves conditioning of some sort) can reject our emotional response, even though this is soul's language. We can prevent this happening by nurturing our emotional growth.

To begin the nurturing process, we need to understand that our emotions are not us – they are a signalling system that tells us where we are in terms of our spiritual development (how clear the line is to soul). But we cannot totally express and create who we really are if our emotional behaviour prevents this. When we are aware of the mental programmes that determine our emotional responses, we can choose to be in control of them. Healing strengthens our emotional life, by drawing our attention to negative mindsets.

Healers Need A Stable Personality

The practice of Sacred Mindfulness emphasizes the importance of relating to our personality and physicality because these are the vehicles for the experiences of soul and the transmission of Love into physical life. This includes our emotional life. Meditation is not a means for rejecting self but of experiencing self as Oneness.

For this reason we see work on ourselves as important in developing a stable personality (ego) and a strong sense of who we are. Healing is an energetic force that will challenge the psychological strength of our personality. A person with a weak or wounded ego will not have the stability needed for grounding and integrating spiritual experiences. Indeed, a powerful spiritual experience may become overwhelming or even destructive for such a person.

When we have addressed our own wounding and the ego is stable, we will be better equipped to experience the emotional upsets life may bring and to sit with the patient's expression of wounding without becoming defensive, limiting the support available and fearful of accompanying the patient as they undertake the journey towards healing and wholeness.

We can greatly strengthen the stability of our emotional response through maintaining the conscious awareness that we have begun to develop through the practice of Sacred Mindfulness. With this in mind, have a look again at Action Points 6 and 7 (in Chapter 5).

ADDRESSING REPRESSED ASPECTS OF SELF

The experience of great healers like Fools Crow is that the condition of the hollow bone (the healing 'channel') is directly related to our personal development and the transformation of destructive ways of thinking and feeling. This means acceptance and respect for our total self, just as we are, without conditions or judgement. The loving, unconditional positive regard that we have for the patient must be extended to ourselves (for we are not separate from them).

As long as we are not prepared to look at repressed aspects of our nature, they will be kept in the shadows of our own created darkness. These happen to be the ideal conditions in which repressed aspects of personality will grow and intensify.

When we are unaware of the emotional energies, mental patterns and habits that lie in the darkness, they are able to emerge, without much warning, to overwhelm, dominate and extinguish our clarity and awareness when emotional conditions are present which can trigger such a response. Whenever this happens, our capacity to consciously choose our behaviour is severely weakened and the mental programme has control.

Repressed aspects of self are not necessarily negative at all, but their emergence at inappropriate moments produces a negative result for us. Every time the soul message conflicts with the distorted mental programme, the emotional energies of the repressed material are released. When this happens, we have identified so closely with the emotional energy that our personality can appear to be transformed in a few moments.

Nigel had found ways to repress most of his emotions and became worried that he could no longer express feelings of tenderness or love for others. He was also disturbed that whenever his mother criticized his way of looking after his business affairs this triggered feelings originally generated by his mother's attitude to him when he was a child. Soon he would be a raging, needy child again. Other people making the same kind of remark would trigger a similar reaction, especially if they were women. After several healing sessions, Nigel became more and more aware of his negative patterns of feeling and behaviour, and began to face them. In this way he was able to identify them, to see how they had been created and to disengage from their dominating hold on his feelings. This opened up his heart so that he could begin to express the emotions that had been missing from his life for so long.

As Nigel's story shows, any process of repression restrains and confines a range of feelings and emotions. These may often contain within them the vital energies of passion, enthusiasm, joy of living and sense of freedom. Sacred Healing sees the repressed aspect of a person as part of their whole being. Through healing, this aspect is released or the patient is shown how to release it so that its vitality is available to energize the patient's transformation towards a healthy integration of self.

With a good grasp of how mind and emotions have influenced our life, we will gain insight into our patient's experience if we look at our own. The next Action Point looks at the training mind has received and the power it holds.

ACTION POINT 27 How Mind Affects the Message

Developmental tool – promoting awareness of mind's role in blocking soul impulse and communication.

This exercise may also be used as a self-healing technique to identify situations where the mind blocks soul impulses – perhaps a pattern may emerge.

- Sit together with a partner and talk about a time you remember when mind talked you out of heeding your soul message. Your partner should listen without commenting.

- Talk about your feelings at the time or any you have had about the subject since.

- What action *did* you take? What was the eventual outcome?

- Your partner shares how it felt to be hearing your story, without giving you advice.

- Change roles and repeat the procedure.

POSITIVE THINKING AND DEALING WITH HEAVY ENERGY

As well as gently persevering with Sacred Mindfulness practice, we can support our emotional growth by working with our mental programmes. While we are doing this, we need to look at our attitudes. These are expressions of our mindsets.

A constructive mental attitude prevents the absorption of heavy energy into the field. Heavy energy is attracted to the depressed, despairing or despondent person, as well as to fear, anger, irritation, argument and complaining.

Clear the field when this happens or if you are in the presence of heavy energy. If allowed to accumulate it will affect a tired or weak part of the body or mind. It is a question of practising recognition and awareness and acting on it.

ACCEPTING THE GIFT OF LIFE

Soul has answered the call of Earth to come here and we have earned the right to be here at this special time during the raising of the consciousness of the planet. Our soul mission is to express the needs of soul and to address the needs of the planet's soul. This begins with accepting the gift of life.

Most of us like some parts of our life and reject the rest, wishing for something different, and we have trained our mind to accept and to reject. We have not realized that when we reject life we reject the Source and we reject ourselves. The eventual suffering involved is a signal of our non-acceptance. The degree of our suffering is the scale that shows us how much we reject the gift of life.

When we reject life, for whatever reason, we also reject the body that is living the life and the senses that tell us we are alive. The body is aware of this through the network of consciousness and through messages it may receive via the energy centres. In extreme circumstances, we may wish to give up our life. This can take the form of suicide or a kind of slow suicide, such as a destructive lifestyle. Or disease may be our way of handing the gift of Earth life back.

Mind does what it is trained to do and we carry on doing the training. Just like a badly trained dog, it can seem to be out of control, working against us, taking on habits, addictions and patterns of self-destructive behaviour. But the 'dog' was allowed to get out of control by its temporary owner, the personality.

Healing enables the true owner of mind, the soul, to exert pressure on us to retrain the mind to assist soul's mission.

The core of soul's mission is to accept whatever life brings, to accept totally the life gift. For in this gift are the challenges that soul wishes to face. So we need to take up life's challenges and work with them, rather than accepting some and rejecting others. This, of course, does not mean that we leave life exactly as it is, but we look at what life is challenging us to do.

HARNESSING THE POWER OF THE MIND

Having seen the destructive power of the mind, we can realize that this is only showing us one side of its great power. We have trained it to be destructive. So we can train our mind to be a powerful ally in creating health and well-being, just as we may have used it in the rejection of some aspects of life.

With spiritual insight, we can see that what was formerly a problem is now an opportunity/challenge. We have an opportunity to see the life of soul as it really is.

Even illness, when realization comes, is an opportunity for growth. Sometimes this is the form of pressure that soul has brought to bear so that there is a breakthrough to the spiritual as a result of the suffering.

During the process of personal transformation, we can create a life way that has built into it constant reminders of our true identity. This is a life way that takes what comes as a gift and works with the challenges, whatever these may be.

These are the insights about life, disease, suffering and acceptance our patients have shared with us in their healing sessions. They show how it is possible to develop a new and healthy relationship with mind and the other systems through which soul operates.

Life is the cosmic gift we carry. All the aspects of being human have equal parts to play in this sacred life. Our body and its faculties are also what we asked for and these are divine gifts too. The body is where the action is, through which soul's creative purpose is carried out. In the next chapter we get to know the body from this point of view.

10

The Travelling Structure

Martin's body had been badly damaged during a car accident. A spinal injury, two broken legs, chest injuries and a broken arm had severly challenged Martin's will to survive. Despite a poor prognosis Martin had struggled hard and learned to walk again. But where was he going? 'Nowhere, fast!' he often joked.

During the healing sessions, Martin questioned the reasons for his accident. Why had he accepted a lift that evening? Why had he survived when his friend had died? Why would he want to experience so much pain? His questions remained unanswered until he was ready to hear his own answers.

The energy scans revealed that the impact upon the travelling structure, his physical body, had sent shock waves throughout Martin's energy system. After a year, healing had helped Martin to restore his mobility and address the emotional and mental trauma of his experience of the accident and the death of his friend.

He continued his healing and gradually the spiritual dynamic of his experience began to impress itself on to Martin's consciousness – he had to change his life – and in a big way.

It had taken a very traumatic experience to act as a wake-up call.

From an unemployed, disillusioned, angry young man already in trouble with the police, and with a drink and drug problem, Martin changed his life around. His wake-up call resulted in a return to studying. Today, seven years later, Martin is a project leader in environmental sciences, working to help communities in drought-affected areas of the world.

Within Spiritual Healing the healer recognizes the possibility that a physical experience, such as an accident or illness, is often a dramatic wake-up call from soul urging the patient to stop, take time out, have a rethink, replan life, take a different direction. The healer also knows that to recover from such experiences and then to carry on as before can be an invitation to another set of traumatic experiences. The soul will be heard.

THE BODY AS A SOUL CREATION

The third aspect of our humanity is the body, which is designed so that the soul can express itself through it. The soul is not confined to the body and it is more accurate to think of soul carrying the body around with it.

The body is the manifestation of a soul need, a spiritual creation with a spiritual and a human function. Problems arise for people when they are unaware of the dual nature of the body and unaware of the soul messages that are being conveyed to it. This is often where the healer comes in when they are asked to 'fix' the physical condition.

Each level of the human being has a human and subtle aspect. Thus, through the mental and emotional 'bodies', we have ways of being conscious of life and of being able to think and feel about it, but our mental and emotional impressions are informed by the material we can sense via the brow and heart centres, which is subtle, intuitive or soul-based. We saw in Chapter 7, The Light Body, how the physical body was created from the etheric and how its organs and systems are derived from etheric structures.

We are going to look at the body from this point of view – that it is a soul creation with a dual purpose. We will see if this view enhances our understanding of how Spiritual Healing is carried out and what effects it might have on the body.

THE CELL — THE FUNDAMENTAL UNIT OF THE BODY

If you could break down all the parts of your body into tiny units, you would find it composed of millions of cells. If these were further broken down into molecules, then atoms, you would end up with the smallest of units, the subatomic particles, all of which are vibrating patterns of energy.

Because energy originates from the Source of consciousness, all energy is conscious to some degree. This has important implications for health and healing, for it follows that each energy pattern will be conscious, whether it is a particle, a cell, an organ or a complete physical body. It also follows that every unit of energy within a large pattern, such as an organ, will be in touch with every other unit of energy through the network of consciousness. Further, what is happening to these physical energies may be transmitted to the mental, emotional and soul levels via etheric consciouness.

In its turn, mind generates thought and this affects the consciousness of the physical energies. This is how thought and feeling influences matter at an energetic level, having a profound effect on the harmony of the body. In this way, energetic influences can alter the behaviour of the body's minutest components, the very energies that go to build its structure and compose its interrelated systems.

The cell is the fundamental unit in all the physical forms of human, animal and plant. Every activity of an organ or a body as a whole happens as a result of the organized and co-ordinated activities of the cells. The nucleus of the cell directs the processes it is designed to carry out, via the information carried in the DNA, and indirectly via messages from the brain. But at a subtle level the nucleus is also directed by etheric consciousness and the supply of the life force. If the life force is withdrawn, as at the time of death, the nucleus behaves in an entirely different way and orders the cessation of cellular activities. This ultimately leads to the breakdown of the cell into its chemical components.

When the cells act together to form tissues and organs, they form the various systems that make up the body. Each of the systems acts in a co-ordinated way to ensure the smooth functioning of the body, just as the structures of the etheric body function as a co-ordinated whole. This co-ordination is soul-directed, for it is the energy of soul that holds all things in place.

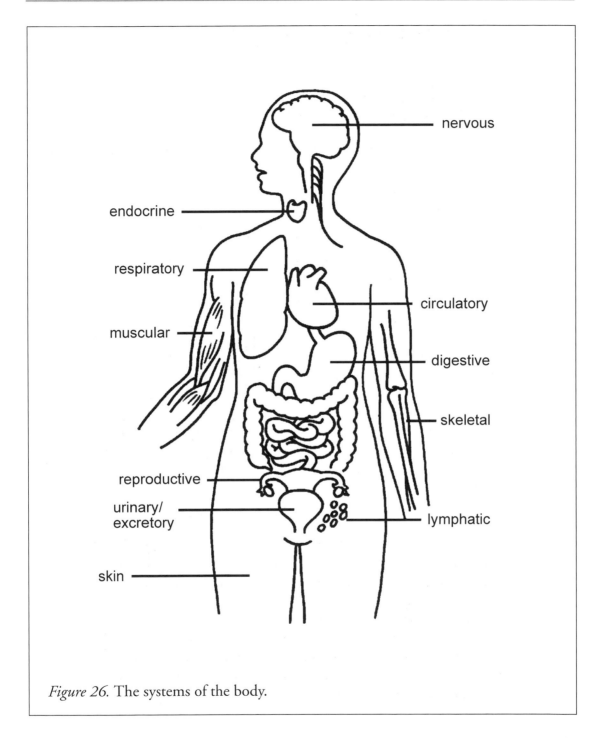

Figure 26. The systems of the body.

THE SKELETON AND ITS SUBTLE ENERGIES

For the body to act as the soul's travelling vehicle, it needs a structure that will provide a strong, rigid, yet highly movable base. This is the physical role of the skeleton. The skeleton has a central flexible column, the spine, which protects the central nervous system. The spine is topped by the skull, which houses and protects the brain. The spine supports two girdles, the shoulders and the pelvis, from which hang the bones of the arms and legs. The rib cage, emanating from the spine and joined in front by the breast bone, houses and protects the heart, lungs, stomach, liver and associated organs. Etheric consciousness is aware of the energetic state of the bones through the subtle energy circuits of the skeleton. The pattern of the energy circuits forms the basis of the second healing scan. In Figure 27, we have indicated the circuits in black for clarity, but they should be thought of as fine lines of light. You can see that the circuits have a central column, which is aligned with the spine with branches at the shoulders and pelvis. These then follow the line of the arms and legs on either side.

The bones also carry information about where a person is on their journey and where that person is situated in terms of the planet. This is why the skeletal energy circuits are scanned so that balance and healing is relayed to these aspects of our being.

THE POLARITY OF THE ENERGY FIELD AND THE SKELETON

The energy circuits of the skeleton reflect the polarity energy channels in the etheric, outlined in Chapter 7, The Light Body. Similarly, the subtle energy circuits of the skeleton are a secondary system whose function is to ensure the balance of energy flow in the skeleton and muscles. Thus, this system is very much associated with the proper movement of the limbs and joints, and the efficient mobility of the whole structure to allow travel.

Just as the polarity channels symbolize the cycle of the energies through the etheric body, the skeletal energy circuits symbolize the cycle of energies in the travelling structure, from stasis to movement to stasis, which continues in all the body systems until the withdrawal of the life force.

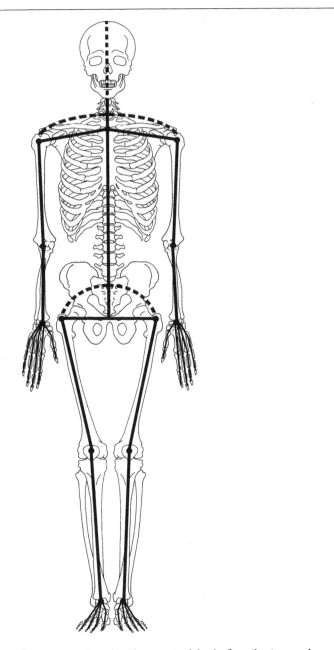

Figure 27. The skeleton with energy circuits shown in black for clarity – they should be visualized as channels of light.

During the healing procedure, the healer works with the balance of the skeletal energy circuits, as well as with the balance of the polarity channels (see if you notice this in Chapter 14, The Sacred Meeting).

ACTION POINT 28 Checking the Balance of the Skeletal Energy Circuit

Developmental tool – promoting awareness of the energetic state of balance within the skeletal energy circuit.

- Your partner should lie on a healing couch. You are standing by your partner's feet. If your partner is seated, squat by your partner's feet and proceed in the same way.

- Hold your palms 5 to 10cm away from the soles of (or above) your partner's feet and sense the energies emanating from them. Do both feet feel the same?

- Does energy *leave* your palms to bring balance so that both feet feel the same energetically?

- Ask your partner what they are aware of.

- Now ask your partner to try to sense the energy leaving your palms to travel up the energy circuits of their legs. What are they aware of?

- Change over and repeat the two procedures.

- Compare notes.

Having established the energetic polarity of the skeleton and energy field, you will understand why the energy circuit scan has to reflect this. The energy circuits of the skeleton are the link between etheric consciousness and the skeleton.

**ACTION POINT 29 Sensing the Skeletal Energy Circuits –
Patient on the Couch**

Developmental tool – promoting awareness of and sensitivity
to energetic material carried by the skeletal energy circuit, using
the energetic structures of the palm.

*This is the basis of the skeletal healing scan. Remember, your intention is to
make contact with the energy circuits of the skeleton, with your palm centres
acting as scanning sensors. First, scan the primary circuit of the spine, then
down one side, scanning the shoulder girdle and arm, the pelvis and leg. Then
down the other side, to balance each of the polarities. The spine is the centre
line as starting point of the secondary circuits. Your partner should lie on the
couch on his back. At all times, follow the form of the skeleton. Since the
instructions for this exercise appear complicated, until practised, it may be helpful to have a third person read them out, or follow a tape.*

- Your partner should relax and breathe normally. You are standing by your
  partner's head. Hold your palms 5 to 10cm above the skull. Move them
  slowly across the skull and down over the face towards the neck, to sense
  where the spine links with the skull. This is where your primary scan of the
  spine begins. Keep one hand at this point while you move the other slowly
  along the spine until you reach its base at the coccyx. Now see if you can feel
  the energy of the spine between your palms.

- To move down the left side of the body, put both palms opposite the base
  of the neck. Your left hand will be the leading hand. Move the left hand
  slowly towards the shoulder, scanning the bones between the neck and the
  shoulder joint. Sense the energy between your palms. Follow with the right
  hand. With both hands at the left shoulder, move the left hand slowly down
  the left arm to the tips of the fingers. Sense the energy between your palms.
  Follow with the right.

- Now scan the left leg. Put your hands opposite the base of the spine. Move
  the left hand across the pelvis to the left hip, scanning the bones of the pelvis.
  Sense the energies between your palms. Follow with the right hand. With

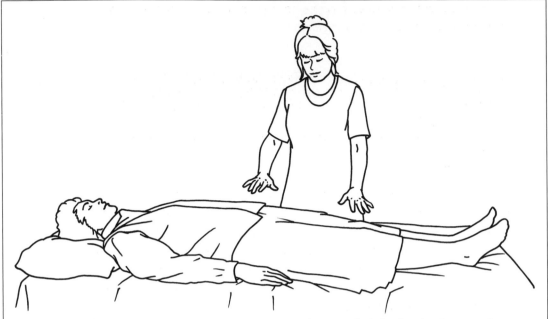

Figure 28. The energy circuit scan, patient on the couch. The healer is scanning from left hip to left knee.

both hands at the left hip, move your left hand slowly down the leg to the toes. Sense the energy between your palms. Follow with the right.

- Now scan the right side. Return your hands to the base of the neck. The right hand is the leading hand. Move the right hand to the right shoulder. Sense as before. Follow with the left. With both hands at the right shoulder, move your right hand slowly down the arm to the tips of the fingers. Sense the energy. Follow with the left hand.

- Return your hands to the base of the spine to scan the right leg. Move your right hand across the pelvis to the right hip. Sense the energies between your palms. Follow with the left.

- With both hands at the right hip, move your hand slowly down the leg to the toes. Sense the energy. Follow with the left. Stand where your partner can see you.

- You have completed your scan of the energy circuits of the skeleton. Discuss your impressions with your partner.

ACTION POINT 30 Sensing the Energy Circuits – Patient on the Chair

Read through the previous Action Point so that you are acquainted with its method and purpose.

- Your partner should relax and breathe normally. Stand behind your partner with your palms held 5 to 10cm away from the back of the skull. Move them slowly down the skull, over the back of the head, towards the neck, until you sense where the spine links with the skull. This is where your primary scan of the spine begins. Keep one hand at this point, while you move the other slowly down the spine until you reach its base at the coccyx. Now see if you can feel the energy of the spine between your palms.

- To move down the left side of the body, put both palms opposite the base of the neck. Your left hand will be the leading hand. Move the left hand slowly towards the shoulder, scanning the bones between the neck and the shoulder joint. Sense the energy between your palms. Follow with the right hand. With both hands at the left shoulder, move the left hand slowly down the left arm to the elbow. Sense the energy betweeen your palms. Follow with the right hand. Move the left hand to the tips of the fingers. Sense the energy between your palms. Follow with the right.

- Now scan the left leg. Put your hands opposite the base of the spine. Move the left across the pelvis to the left hip, scanning the bones of the pelvis. Sense the energies between your palms. Follow with the right hand. With both hands at the left hip, move your left hand slowly down the leg to the knee. Sense the energy between your palms. Follow with the right hand. Move your left hand to the ankle. Sense the energy between your palms. Follow with the right hand. Move your left hand across the foot to the toes. Sense the energy between your palms. Follow with the right.

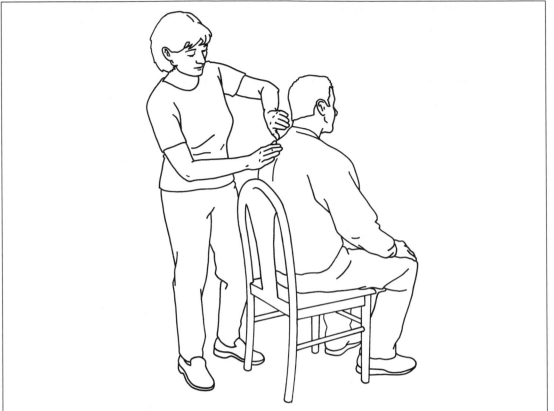

Figure 29. The energy circuit scan, patient on the chair. The healer is scanning the patient's spine.

- Now scan the right side. Return your hands to the base of the neck. The right hand is the leading hand. Move the right hand to the right shoulder. Sense as before. Follow with the left. With both hands at the right shoulder, move your right hand slowly down the arm to the elbow. Sense as before. Follow with the left. Move your right hand to the tips of the fingers. Sense the energy. Follow with the left hand.

- Return your hands to the base of the spine to scan the right leg. Move your right hand across the pelvis to the right hip. Sense the energies between your palms. Follow with the left. With both hands at the right hip, move your hand slowly down the leg to the knee. Sense the energy. Follow with the left. Move your right hand to the ankle. Sense the energy. Follow with the right. Move your right hand across the foot to the toes. Sense the energy. Follow with the left.

- Stand where your partner can see you. You have completed your scan of the energy circuits of the skeleton. Discuss your impressions with your partner.

When you come to carry out the skeletal healing scan as part of the healing procedure, you will notice that it is amplified to make it more thorough (see Chapter 14, The Sacred Meeting).

GATEWAYS FROM THE ETHERIC TO THE PHYSICAL – THE ENDOCRINE GLANDS

The physical gateways for the energies of the main etheric centres are the endocrine glands, the glands without ducts. Their function is linked to the life issues of the relevant centres.

The endocrine system transmits chemical messages in the form of hormones carried in the bloodstream to affect a particular organ or organs. The numerous functions of the glands are their physical role, but they also receive a range of subtle energies, via the etheric centres, which have a direct effect on these functions.

The relationship between the centres and the endocrine glands

The *adrenal glands*, at the top of the kidneys, control the balance of salt in the body fluids and help prepare the body for emergencies and stress through the secretion of adrenaline. This is the link of survival and physical life with the *base centre*.

The *testes* in males control sexual development and maturity and the production of sperm. The *ovaries* in females control sexual development and maturity and the production of eggs. These are the creative links with the *sacral* centre.

The *Islets of Langerhans* in the *pancreas* are groups of endocrine cells. These produce a range of hormones, among which is insulin, the controller

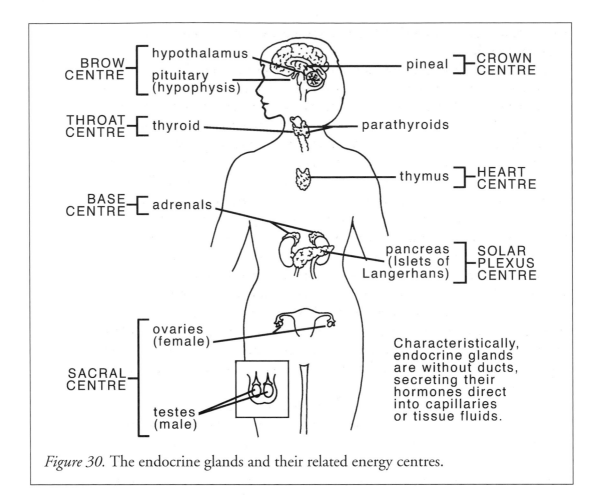

Figure 30. The endocrine glands and their related energy centres.

of the blood sugar level. The secretions of these hormones are linked to the functions of the *solar plexus centre*. Through its link with mind and emotions, our thoughts and feelings have a powerful effect on this gland and the neighbouring organs.

The *thymus gland* is closely related to the development and function of the body's immune system. In the baby it is relatively very large. In childhood it controls the production of white blood cells and the 'T' lymphocytes of the lymphatic system. Though its activities may not appear to be important in the adult, the thymus gland is directly influenced by the energies of the *heart centre*. Practice shows that this centre continues to have a profound influence on the immune system, via the thymus gland, throughout life. There is therefore a strong connection between the state of love in our life and our immune health.

The *thyroid gland* controls the rate of metabolism and body growth. Embedded in the thyroid are the parathyroids, which control the level of calcium in the blood and so have a relationship with the skeleton and teeth. These glands are directly influenced by the energies of the *throat centre*. This centre also affects the ear, nose and throat, via the thyroid gland.

The *hypothalamus* is the main controller of the *pituitary gland* and the endocrine system and monitors all information about body states. This controlling aspect of the pituitary gland is a mirror of some of the functions of the *brow centre* to which it is linked. The pituitary gland is the main controller of the activities of the nervous and endocrine systems (the two control systems of the body), and acts as an intermediary between the body and the brain. The brow centre also co-ordinates the activities of the centres and the system of etheric channels and meridians. The hypothalamus communicates with the pituitary either by nervous impulses or by its own hormones. These, in turn, stimulate the pituitary to secrete a range of hormones, which affect most of the body's functions, through the stimulation of other glands and organs. Thus, all of the body's functions are affected by the energies of the brow centre.

The *pineal gland* lies behind and above the hypothalamus. It is sensitive to light. As daylight fades to darkness, the pineal gland secretes the hormone melatonin. As daylight returns secretion stops. During the winter months, melatonin secretion is higher than in summer. In this way, the pineal gland acts as a light sensor, informing the body of the rhythm of day and night and the passing of the seasons. It is the topmost gland of the endocrine system. It is affected by light and it talks to us about light. This is its link with the *crown centre*, the place where the Light enters our subtle energy system.

Effects of the subtle energies on the body

Because of their interconnectedness, what happens to us physically has an energetic effect that is conveyed to the etheric centres and, if necessary, to the emotional and/or mental levels. Similarly, energies from these levels move to the physical to be processed in this form.

When energies from the soul, mental and emotional levels move into the body, via the endocrine system, they first affect the organs associated with

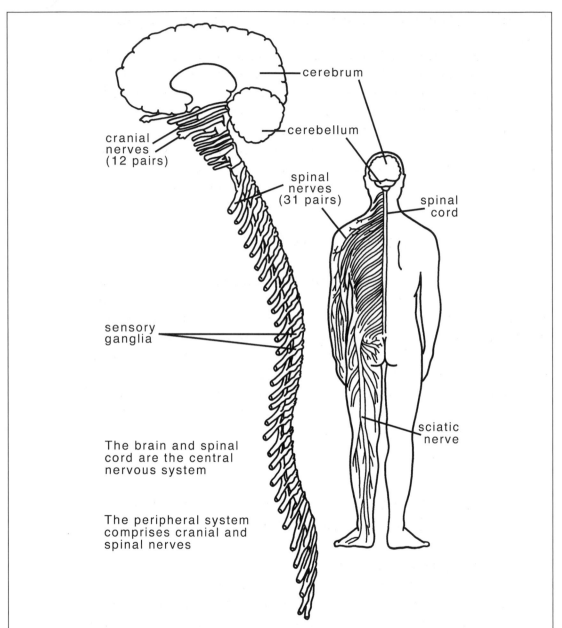

Figure 31. The central nervous system, showing the brain, spinal cord, and spinal nerves. All other nerves are branches, or secondary and tertiary branches of the main structure.

the particular gland and then move further to affect related organs and systems.

For example, the death of a loved one may impact on the heart centre. The energetic implications of the loss are conveyed to the thymus gland and thence to the immune system, so that the person becomes prone to catch a cold, etc. But the effects may go further to influence other parts of the immune system, such as the lymphatic, spleen and tonsils. The person may try to deal with their loss by suppressing the energies generated in the heart centre, encouraging the effects to move further – to the physical heart, the lungs and the bronchial area, even to the upper arms and shoulders.

THE NERVOUS SYSTEM

Most of the control and communication that goes on in the body is carried out by the nervous system. Its messages are transmitted by means of electro-chemical impulses, with the brain acting as the command centre. The extensive network of nerves branching from the spinal cord allows the brain to keep in touch with all the other body systems and to process everything that is happening to us internally and externally.

These are the physical functions of the nervous system. The light aspect of the system is to gather up the messages of the network of consciousness and convey them to the etheric level and thence to the centres, via the etheric network of channels.

THE BLOOD SYSTEM – THE FOURTH SUPPORT SYSTEM OF THE BODY

The organs and systems of the body need oxygen and nutrients to function properly. These life-sustaining materials are carried to every cell via the flow of blood throughout the body. The flow is maintained by the heart, a muscular organ that acts like a pump. Arteries carry oxygenated blood to the cells and away from the heart. The veins carry all blood to the heart. This is the system's physical function.

The ancients treated blood with great respect. It is certain that many groups also knew of the light aspect of its work. The body has four subtle

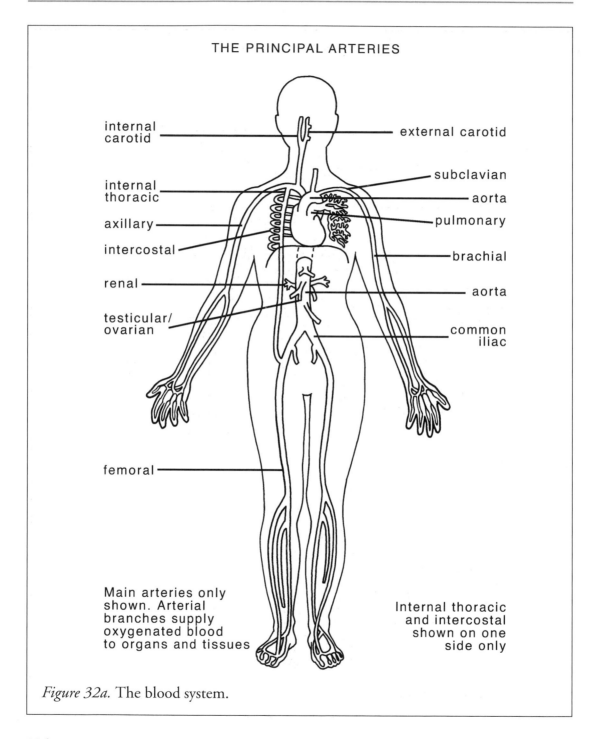

THE PRINCIPAL ARTERIES

internal carotid

external carotid

internal thoracic

subclavian

aorta

axillary

pulmonary

intercostal

renal

brachial

testicular/ ovarian

aorta

common iliac

femoral

Main arteries only shown. Arterial branches supply oxygenated blood to organs and tissues

Internal thoracic and intercostal shown on one side only

Figure 32a. The blood system.

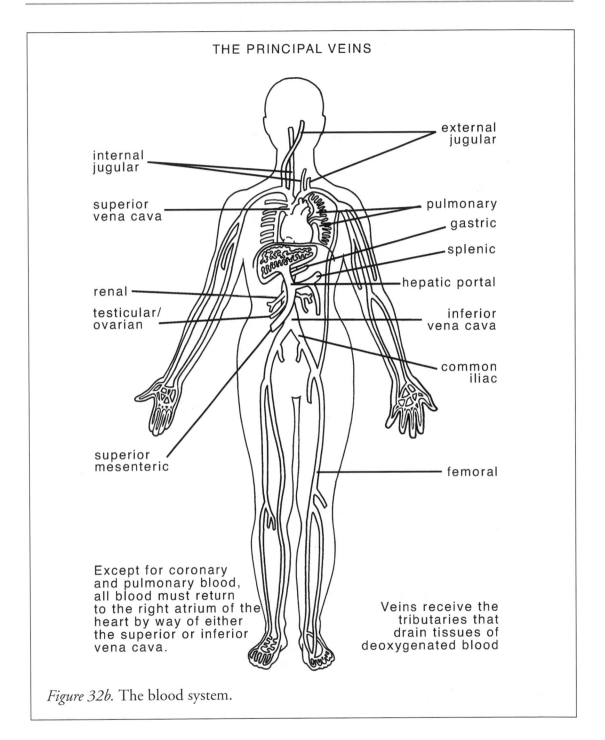

THE PRINCIPAL VEINS

external jugular

internal jugular

superior vena cava

renal

testicular/ ovarian

superior mesenteric

pulmonary

gastric

splenic

hepatic portal

inferior vena cava

common iliac

femoral

Except for coronary and pulmonary blood, all blood must return to the right atrium of the heart by way of either the superior or inferior vena cava.

Veins receive the tributaries that drain tissues of deoxygenated blood

Figure 32b. The blood system.

support systems. These are the etheric, the endocrine, the nervous and the vascular (blood). The subtle energies of the first three are transported by the bloodstream, which is derived from the *flow* of energy within the etheric network. As we mentioned earlier, the blood carries the life force to every cell and this function is also derived from the modifications of the light body.

When any part of this support system is stressed or in danger of breaking down, the body is able to draw attention to it. Because of this we can guarantee that, no matter how much we have to focus on other people's bodies, we will not be allowed to forget our own.

As we have seen already, looking after your body is part of the healer's responsibility to yourself and your patients. But the body also speaks to us about familiarity and friendship. We can be a fair-weather friend to our body where we only remember it when it finds a discomforting way of pointing out any disharmony in the system.

This is why some sort of exercise is essential to maintain the friendship. See exercise as a way of spending quality time with yourself and a way of showing love and consideration to this aspect of soul. Exercise allows you to get to know your body.

And now consider how well you know your hands.

HANDS

You may need to become reacquainted with your hands. All these years you have been using them to do so many thousands of tasks that it is difficult to imagine life without them. Along with language, the use of the hand, with its fingers and thumb, is said to exemplify the human. But you also have been living with the subtle energetic aspect of your hands, which is their energy centres and their link with the heart centre and the expression or denial of Love. This link is so powerful that when the hands are used to do unloving things, such as hurt another, the centres of the palms and the heart register this as abuse.

Have a look at your hands, slowly scanning them on both sides. Relax your body and relax your vision, and see if you become aware in some way of the tremendous energy exchanges that go on in the hands. As well as the subtle energies, a number of physical energies radiate from the hands, especially the fingertips, which can be photographed with modern Kirlian-type cameras (see Glossary).

Allow your hands to speak to you – in them is the story of your life. You grew your hands in your mother's womb and while still there you got to know the feel of them by moving them about, and opening and closing them. You found that you could touch parts of your own body. A contemplation and meditation on your hands will be richly rewarding.

The body demonstrates the intention to help another by the reaching out of the hands. This the mind knows. The history of 'hands-on' healing and the beginning of care probably goes back to the time of the first humans – all because of the energy link between the hands and the heart. Most of us are out of touch with this link, but healers need to strengthen it – even if your way of working is through distant healing.

Every time you reach to help, comfort or console another being, you strengthen the hand-heart link. Of course any healing work will do the same. But we cannot do too much to create the hollow bone.

The next Action Point will keep your hands at a high level of sensitivity for healing and allow the contact of your hands with the things in your life to be moments of meditation (being with Oneness) and give you great pleasure.

ACTION POINT 31 Strengthening the Hand-Heart Link

Developmental tool – promoting sensitivity to energy communication channels between the heart and palms.

This exercise may also be used as a self-healing technique for expressing Love through the hands. It opens the heart centre and activates the palm centres.

- Gather a number of objects in front of you. Relax and focus on your hands. Breathe gently into the palms, breathing the energy up your arms, across the shoulders to the heart centre. After a few breaths, relax and breathe normally.

- Pick up an object and fondle it as if you feel great love for it. Realize that it is composed of the energy of the Source, like all other matter. You are able to caress Oneness. Your hands put you in contact with the energy of Oneness in a special way. How does it feel? Do the same with the other objects.

- Use the same procedure and attitude to touch the place where you live, the walls, the ground, the air, the water.

- Extend your experiencing to plants and animals – a leaf, flower, the bark of a tree, the fur of a dog, etc.

- Finally, when you have experienced all this range of sensations and awarenesses, find some humans to touch in the same way!

- Your hands will remember these directed experiences. Allow them to come to mind when you go to give healing.

SUBTLE ASPECTS OF FOOD

Living things need feeding if they are not to begin deteriorating. The digestive system, like all the other bodily systems, works at a subtle as well as a physical level with the food and drink we consume.

The physical function of digestion begins in the mouth through the interaction of saliva with the food. The subtle level of digestion also begins here with the finest vibrations of the food being absorbed by the tongue. The body needs the subtle aspects of food and drink, and will find ways of alerting us if it does not get enough in quality and quantity, or if it is getting too much!

The longer the food remains in the mouth, the more benefit you will obtain from the two levels of digestion.

What does your body think about rushing to eat, eating without caring what you put in your mouth, eating for the sake of eating? Have you ever asked it? Well, there's another meal coming up soon!

Because food has been part of a living plant or animal, it contains a range of vibrations. Blessing your food thanks it, clears it and brings its energies into alignment with your own.

ACTION POINT 32 Blessing Food

Developmental tool – using the hands in a sacred manner to enhance the energy structures of the palms.

This exercise may also be used as a self-healing exercise to assess the compatability of food and drink. It is also an opportunity to give thanks to the plants, animals and mineral kingdom that provide food and to those who have prepared it.

- When you are going to eat something, first hold your hands over the food to see if your body really needs it. If you sense that it does not, honour your intuitve awareness by not consuming the food.

- All food can be honoured through your remembrance of the hand-heart link. Use your hands to bless and thank your food and drink when you are going to consume them.

Getting together, celebrating and eating with others is a wonderful way of sharing food. Your emotions tell you all this. Food should always be eaten with enjoyment and never with anxiety about what it is made of. Blessing your food has already taken care of this, so go ahead and enjoy your food as a gift from the planet. Thank those who prepare it for you. When this is just not possible, do it mentally.

The Action Points in this chapter will help you to understand the physical body, its structures and functions, as an expression of etheric/soul consciousness.

We move on now to another vital system, which, like all the body systems, functions on behalf of the human and the light body. This is the respiratory system that allows us to take in air, oxygen and the life force through the breath. As we shall see, it has a close relationship with our ability or inability to relax.

The Tools of
Spiritual Healing

11

Sacred Tools:
Breathing and Relaxation

THE GIFT OF CONSCIOUS BREATHING

Apart from the gift of presence, the healer offers patients gifts of empowerment, which they can use during healing sessions and in the course of their own lives. Anything that empowers the patient enhances the healing session and effectively becomes a healing tool – something that has a special role in healing. The first of the sacred tools of healing is the gift of conscious breathing.

Unless we suffer from a respiratory disorder, such as asthma, we do not have to think about our breathing. Just like the blood circulation, it is automatic, under the control of the autonomic nervous system. Like the other systems of the body, such as the endocrine glands, we do not have to ask our breathing apparatus to keep going, since it is a function of the co-ordinated living body. But, as you have seen in some of the Action Points earlier, we can intervene to control our breathing in a beneficial way.

When we are upset, breathing rate and heartbeat increase due to the secretion of adrenaline. By controlling our breathing and calming it, we can regain the balance of mind and emotions. This sends a message to the adrenal glands to stop secreting adrenaline so that breath and heartbeat are further calmed.

By the simple act of controlling our breathing, we are better able to cope. So breathing will be one of the first things the healer notices about the state of the patient on arrival.

Most of us do not breathe properly and use only a small part of the lungs, often due to factors such as stress, bad posture and lack of exercise. We can change the bad habit of inefficient breathing by short, but regular, sessions of conscious breathing.

HOW BREATHING WORKS

The diaphragm, the large muscle forming the floor of the chest, at the base of the rib cage, is creating the condition we call breathing. When the

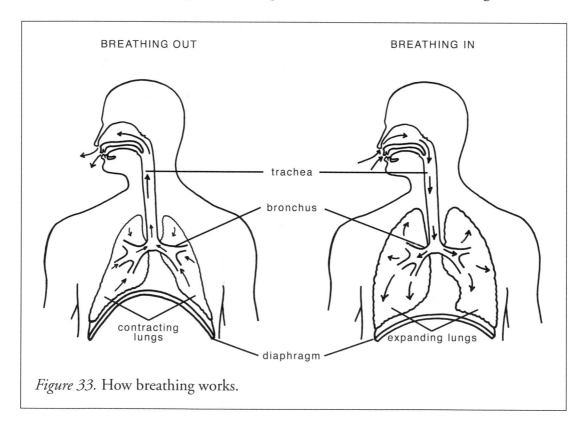

Figure 33. How breathing works.

diaphragm is flattened downwards, the cavity enclosed by the rib cage is enlarged, creating a vacuum. The lungs are suspended in this cavity and immediately expand to fill the space, drawing in air via the nose or mouth. The diaphragm then relaxes upwards, which deflates the lungs, forcing the breath to be expelled.

There are thus two breaths, the in-breath and the out-breath, both of which you may feel as different sensations. As air is breathed into the lungs, oxygen passes through their fine membranes into the bloodstream to oxygenate the cells and tissues. As you exhale, waste gases, such as carbon dioxide, leave the bloodstream to be expelled.

THE SUBTLE ROLE OF BREATHING

That is the basic physical function of breathing. But it also has a light body function, which is to carry the life force (*prana* or *qi*) and information from etheric consciousness to every part of the physical, via the blood system. This ability to carry subtle energies means that the patient is able to take in healing energies from the energy field, set up during the healing session, through conscious breathing (see Chapter 14, The Sacred Meeting).

The breath of life is indeed more than breathing in and out. When the newborn baby takes its first breath it is a great affirmation of the role of air as carrier of oxygen and, just as importantly, carrier of the life force and etheric consciousness. Just as the in-breath is a way of taking in what we need, the out-breath is a signal for energy to escape. Anything that needs to escape, to be released or to find a way out of the system, can do so on the out-breath. When you are using breath in this way, to let go of stress or anxiety, for example, it is helpful to do so with the open mouth since this reminds you that your conscious out-breath has this function — you can also do so with more force if necessary.

In the following Action Point we will practise conscious breathing with its dual role in mind:

ACTION POINT 33 Full Breath Breathing

Developmental tool – promoting increased facility within the physical body to receive and give life through the breath and raising awareness of the sacred nature of breath and breathing.

This exercise may also be used as a self-healing activity to improve breathing capacity and to benefit the whole physical system.

*(**Note:** Anyone experiencing breathing difficulties should only undertake breathing exercises under supervision.)*

This exercise should be taped or read out to you by a partner.

- Sit comfortably with your feet flat on the floor. Notice your breathing. Allow it to become slow, deep and gentle.

- Notice what your chest and abdomen are doing. In full breath breathing, the focus is on the movement of the abdomen, rather than the chest. Put your hands there and imagine it is a balloon you are going to fill and then empty.

- As you slowly inhale through the nose, allow your 'balloon' to fill by letting your abdomen gently swell. Do not strain.

- Exhale slowly and feel the balloon of your abdomen deflate. Again, do not strain.

- Do this exercise three times. Note the difference between the in-breath and the out-breath. Note how you feel as you breathe like this.

The next time you see a sleeping baby, notice the way the baby breathes. How different is this to the way you breathe? Full breath breathing is also known as 'soft-belly breathing' because it encourages the relaxation of the abdomen and discourages the tense, hard-belly approach to body posture. Breathing and posture affect our mood and attitude. They can affect both in a positive way. The soft-belly posture allows you to breathe deeply and gently so that you are calm and balanced, with your centre of gravity below your navel.

The next Action Point extends the technique of full breath breathing to encourage expansion of the lungs and a steady rhythm to the breathing cycle. It can help the patient to realize that it is possible to gain this level of control quite simply and opens the mind to the possibility of empowerment in other areas.

ACTION POINT 34 Rhythmic Breathing

Developmental tool – preparing the respiratory system to give, receive and await the arrival of the sacred impulse between breaths.

This exercise may also be used as a self-healing activity to promote efficient breathing and to affirm the 'I am'.

Tape this exercise or have a partner read it out to you. Sit in the same way as you did for Action Point 33.

- Practise full breath breathing for three complete breaths.

- Now inhale to the count of three. Hold for the count of one. Exhale to the count of three. Hold for the count of one. Do this for three breath cycles.

- See if you can inhale to the count of four. Hold for the count of two. Exhale to the count of four. Hold for the count of two. Breathe to this rhythm for six breaths. Do not strain.

- As you grow relaxed and confident with the four/two rhythm, see if you can increase it to six/three without straining.

- Within the pause between breaths lies all potential, all possibility, everything you are needing at this time. Within the pause is the 'I am'.

Andrea was very nervous about a forthcoming interview. Healing had helped her in the past to face potentially stressful situations. She was reminded of rhythmic breathing. Within the pause between breaths she connected to her confidence and state of calmness. She found the 'I am' and within the 'I am' there was no place for nervousness, fear, or anxiety – they did not exist.

Andrea practised rhythmic breathing daily for two weeks before the interview. It all went well and she was successful in achieving a much prized career move.

ACTION POINT 35 The Rise and Fall of the Breath

Developmental tool – charting body consciousness of life rhythm; regulating life rhythm.

This exercise may also be used as a self-healing activity.
This may be carried out on its own or after either Action Point 33 or 34.

- Sit comfortably as before with your feet flat on the ground, breathing normally.

- As you breathe, notice the rise and fall of your belly for a few moments. Relax into your own rhythm of rise and fall as you inhale and exhale.

- Think of the rise and fall of your belly as the rise and fall of your life experiences. But, just as you can witness the rise and fall of your belly during breathing, so you can witness the ups and downs of your life in the same way. This is the experience of your personality, but you do not have to define yourself by the ups and downs of your life. You are the silent, compassionate witness.

RELAXATION

You will have noticed that, in many of the Action Points so far, conscious breathing and conscious relaxation were important features in preparing yourself to carry them out. Conscious relaxation, the second sacred tool of healing, goes hand in hand with conscious breathing.

Relaxation relieves tension and stress and allows the body energies to flow more freely. The activities of the brain, heart and lungs are slowed down, calming the mind and emotions. This creates the ideal state for healing and meditation.

Many people do not know how to relax and you may need to teach your patients how to do it. The following exercise is a simple, yet thorough method of relaxing the whole body. In it you send a command to the brain to allow all the muscles of the body to relax, release and let go. You co-ordinate this with slow, deep and gentle breathing, which immediately sends positive messages to all the body systems that things are becoming calm and peaceful.

ACTION POINT 36 Full Body Relaxation

Developmental tool – addressing the needs of the physical body; learning to honour the physical vehicle by communicating love for it via relaxation.

This exercise may also be used as a self-healing activity to promote a sense of peace and well-being throughout the physical body.

This Action Point should be taped or read out to you by a partner. Ideally, you should lie on a firm, even surface with a comfortable support for the head and neck.

- Allow your legs to part and move your hands away from the sides of your body.

- Carry out the full breath as in Action Point 33. Breathe slowly, gently and normally.

- Now focus on your hands. Clench them tightly and then let them slowly unclench with the out-breath. Remember the feeling of unclenching (relaxing) and letting go as you exhale. Do not clench anything again throughout the rest of this exercise. As you breathe, know that you are breathing in peace and relaxation. Let any anxieties or problems go with the out-breath; breathe them out through the open mouth.

- Now focus on the toes of your left foot. Feel them relax, one by one. Move slowly over your foot, relaxing the muscles. Let the ankle go. Use the out-breath to let go, release and relax.

- Move up your left leg, relaxing the muscles. Let the knee joint go. Relax the thigh muscles and the muscles of the buttocks.

- Let go across the pelvis. Continue to breathe slowly and gently.

- Focus on your right foot and proceed in the same way, over the foot and up the right leg, slowly and deliberately relaxing and letting go.

- Relax the pelvis again.

- Now come up the front of the body, relaxing the belly and stomach. Let go of the muscles of the chest. Let go of the shoulders.

- Return to the lower back and slowly relax your back muscles, letting them go one by one. Make sure you take time to relax them all if you suffer from lower back pain. Pay attention to the muscles across the top of the back and shoulders where tension also gathers. Relax and let go.

- Relax the left shoulder and move down the left arm. Let the elbow joint go. Move down the forearm, relaxing and letting go. Let the wrist relax.

- Relax the palm, thumb and fingers, one by one.

- Return to the right shoulder. Relax it and move down the right arm in the same way as the left. Relax the whole of the shoulder girdle.

- Now move up your neck, very slowly, relaxing and letting go. Come up the back of the head and over the top of the scalp, relaxing and letting go of all the tiny muscles.

- Imagine a caring hand smoothing your forehead. Relax the eyes, the cheeks, the mouth. Relax the jaw.

- Continue to breathe slowly, gently and normally. Scan your body to see if any part has tensed up again. If it has, relax it, enjoying the feeling of total relaxation. You can remain mentally alert or allow yourself to drift off into sleep.

When you repeat this exercise, try starting the relaxation at the top of the head and making your way down to your toes, using the same technique. See which method is most comfortable for you. If you find it helps you to relax, you might like to put on some quiet, soothing music. Practise relaxation so that it becomes second nature and you can do it anywhere, in any circumstances and in any position.

As well as being an essential requirement in healing, relaxation *is* healing, for the act of letting go allows your energies to come back into balance.

MENTAL RELAXATION

Just as the body needs to be consciously relaxed, so does the mind. This is your second relaxation strategy and it is particularly necessary with a patient whose mind interferes with the healing process or who finds it difficult to mentally relax. The technique is to talk your patient through a gentle trip to a place where they can relax and be at peace, such as beside a beautiful tree or gently flowing stream. Care has to be taken to select imagery that is relaxing for the patient and not confusing. This could happen, for example, if you ask them to visualize walking in the mountains and they have no visual experience of this and/or they would not find it relaxing to do so.

The steps of the journey should always be retraced, going back through the same gates or over the same bridge. In this work, imagery should always be positive and soothing. Bear in mind that, during any relaxation exercise, the patient needs to raise their consciousness.

It can be very effective simply to ask your partner to go to a place where they feel at peace. Later they can tell you what that place was like.

Here is a simple guided visualization to aid mental relaxation that will suit some people. Notice that the scene is set in a European landscape and should be adapted to suit individual needs.

ACTION POINT 37 Mental Relaxation

Developmental tool – honouring the creative role of mind; loving mind through relaxation.

This exercise may also be used for self-healing as an antidote to the effect of daily life stresses.

Lie or sit comfortably. Relax your whole body, as you did in Action Point 36 above, and breathe normally. Your partner should take care to give you time to create each image for yourself and to act on it mentally.

- With eyes closed, see yourself walking along a country lane. It is a warm day and you can feel a slight breeze against your cheeks.

- You feel at peace with yourself and with the world. It seems that everything you see as you walk along increases your feelings of peace and well-being.

- You notice the tiny flowers by the wayside and the sound of the birds in the hedgerows. The air is good to breathe, with the faint scent of plants.

- Up ahead you see a little gate with trees on either side. You open the gate and find yourself in a large, beautiful garden. You see a seat and make your way to it and sit down to rest in these peaceful surroundings. You notice the different flowers. Birds sing in the trees. You feel the peace and beauty of the garden deep inside you. Stay a while to enjoy it. (Allow your partner to remain in the state of mental relaxation for a few minutes.)

- Now it is time to go. You may want to say goodbye to the garden, knowing that you can come back any time you wish.

- Make your way to the gate between the trees, go through and close the gate behind you.

- Walk back down the lane at an easy pace. You recognize some of the plants and bushes as you pass.

- Soon you have made your way back to where you are now. Open your eyes when you feel ready. Become aware of your body lying on the couch/sitting on the chair. Feel your feet.

- Share your experience with your partner. In the learning scenario, change over and talk your partner through a mentally relaxing trip. Again, share the experience.

Begin building a database of relaxing scenarios for use with patients or for yourself. This may be from direct experience or from pictures, postcards, illustrations from favourite works of art, and so on.

BREATHING AND RELAXATION AS HEALING TOOLS

We now move from a physical view of breathing and relaxation to their use as the sacred tools of healing. The following Action Points combine relaxation of the body and mind with conscious breathing.

ACTION POINT 38 Basic Breathing and Relaxation for Healing

Developmental tool – working with the breath to induce a state of relaxation; preparing the energy field to receive healing energies.

This exercise may also be used for self-healing to build upon the body's potential to self-heal through relaxation.

You should be lying supine on a couch. Your partner should talk you through the exercise or you could tape it, leaving pauses where necessary.

- Let yourself relax and breathe normally. Close your eyes and go within. Focus on your breath and your breathing.

- Feel your body breathing. Be aware of your breath entering and leaving your body. Enjoy the feeling of your body breathing. Feel your body moving in time with your breathing. Feel your chest and abdomen responding to your breathing.

- Imagine now that, as you inhale, you can take in all the healing energy you need. And as you breathe out, your body is finding a way of letting go, releasing any stored energy you no longer need. Breathe in to nourish yourself. Breathe out to let go.

- Feel yourself relaxing against the couch and the pillow with every out-breath.

- Now allow your body to find its own breathing rhythm.

- Your body will continue to take in all the energy it needs and to release on the out-breath. Spend a few moments in this healing state.

- Change over and compare notes.

This exercise can stand alone or be used to begin every healing session, or it can be combined with the full relaxation procedure if this is appropriate.

Because of its calming effect on the body, mind and emotions, Action Point 38 usually leads to a deeply relaxed state in the patient. Remember, the more calm and relaxed the patient is, the more they are able to access the healing energy being made available.

The next Action Point goes further to engage the patient in their own healing.

ACTION POINT 39 Using Basic Breathing as an Empowerment Technique

Developmental tool – using the breath to direct energy throughout the physical body.

This exercise may also be used as a self-healing activity.

You are lying supine on the couch, relaxed and breathing normally as for Action Point 38. Your partner should talk you through the exercise or you could tape it, leaving pauses where necessary.

- Close your eyes and go within. Bring your attention to your breath and your breathing. Feel your body breathing.

- Notice your breath entering and leaving your body. Enjoy your body breathing and the movement of your body breathing on your behalf. See yourself taking in all the healing energy you need at this time.

- Breathe in, taking in everything you need. Breathe out, sending the energy down your body, filling your abdomen.

- Breathe in. Breathe out, sending the energy to fill the whole of your pelvis.

- Breathe in. Breathe out, helping the energy to travel down your legs. (You may need several breaths to fill your legs and to reach your feet and toes.)

- Breathe in. Breathe out, filling your chest and shoulders.

- Breathe in. Breathe out, sending the energy down your arms to fill your hands and fingers.

- Breathe in. Breathe out, sending the energy to your throat and neck and up to fill your head.

- Relax your breathing now. Let it find its own rhythm.

- Imagine yourself filled with new energy. Your body will continue breathing in and taking in all the healing energy it needs and breathing out, sending it to where it is needed.

- Change over and talk your partner through the exercise.

Make sure that you match the instructions to the patient's breathing. They may need several breaths for each instruction so it is important to give them plenty of time.

The next Action Point may be used to further empower your patient.

ACTION POINT 40 Breathing in Love, Peace and Light

Developmental tool – linking with the energies of Love, Peace and Light; using the breath to convey energy to the physical via the total energy field.

This exercise may also be used for self-healing.

You are lying supine on the couch, relaxed and breathing normally as for the Action Points above. Your partner should talk you through the exercise or you could tape it, leaving pauses where necessary.

- Close your eyes and go within. Focus on your breath and your breathing. Feel your body breathing. Enjoy the movement of your body breathing.

- See yourself taking in all the healing energy you need at this time.

- We can think of healing energy as made up of Love, Peace and Light. As you inhale, see yourself taking in all the Love you need at this time and fill your body with Love. As you breathe out, send Love into the space around you.

- Again, as you inhale, see yourself taking in all the Peace you need at this time and fill your body with Peace. As you breathe out, send Peace into the space around you.

- On the next in-breath, see yourself taking in all the Light you need at this time and fill your body with Light. As you breathe out, send Light into the space around you.

- Imagine your body now filled with Love, Peace and Light. Feel your body filled with Love, Peace and Light. Feel the space around you filled with Love, Peace and Light.

- Stay within this state for a few moments.

- Change over and talk your partner through the exercise.

In this exercise, the patient is beginning to learn how to work with their own energy field.

Some patients find it helpful to see these aspects of healing energy as colours. Love is often seen as a pink or green light, Peace as blue or white and Light may be white. Your patient may see them all as different colours. Just mentally record this. It may prove indicative of a healing need.

ACTION POINT 41 Attuning to Love, Peace and Light

Developmental tool – working with the energies of Love, Peace and Light via the breath and colour vibrations.

This exercise may also be used for self-healing.

A variation of Action Point 40, when combined with relaxation, is also very suitable to begin your healing procedure. You are lying supine on the couch, relaxed and breathing normally. This exercise could also be used with a seated patient. Your partner should talk you through the exercise or you could tape it, leaving pauses where necessary.

- Close your eyes and go within. Focus on your breath and your breathing. Feel your body breathing and enjoy the movement of your body breathing.

- Some people describe the energy of healing as Love. Allow yourself to breathe in Love and see if a colour appears. Fill your body with this colour.

- Some people describe the energy of healing as Peace. Allow yourself to breathe in Peace and see if a colour appears. Fill your body with this colour.

- Some people describe the energy of healing as Light. Allow yourself to breathe in Light and see if a colour appears. Fill your body with this colour.

- Imagine your body filled with the coloured energies of Love, Peace and Light. Feel the space around you filled with the colours of Love, Peace and Light.

- Change over and talk your partner through the exercise.

In this exercise, the patient is effectively putting themselves in a state of attunement and choosing the type of healing energy they need at that time (as demonstrated by the energy colours). Patients may experience the different colours travelling to specific body areas. Mentally record this — it may prove relevant later in the healing session.

Before using any of the Action Points in your healing session, practise them with a partner and compare notes. In the healing session they should be used intuitively after you have assessed your patient's needs or according to soul guidance. Be sure that you feel confident to give breathing and relaxation instructions in a calm and relaxed manner. Make your own tape and listen to your own voice.

BREATHING AND RELAXATION LEADING TO HEALING STATES

In practice, Action Points 39, 40 and 41 should be introduced session by session as the patient is able to relax, so that each completed exercise builds on the one before.

We have found that the combination of breathing and relaxation in the exercises leads to a number of healing states. Patients choose, at a soul level, which state they need at a particular time.

Total body awareness and rebuilding body relationship

Patients can become totally aware of their bodies. For many this will be a new state of awareness that is both empowering and healing. Patients are often disconnected from their bodies through pain or trauma and need to be reconnected with them. Others may need to be encouraged to build a new relationship with their bodies, especially after surgery. Bodies respond to love and respect.

The patient is guided to experience relaxation as a state of being, as a way of practising being, in which there is nothing to think of, nothing to worry about, nothing to do except simply be.

The 'healing sleep' and its features

There is a relaxation state between total wakefulness and sleeping where patients can go to places where they are completely relaxed and at ease with themselves.

Some patients may move into what we call a 'healing sleep'. In this state they can leave their body and move into the so-called astral body (the vehicle soul uses for travelling out of the physical body) to facilitate the healing. The patient may, or may not, return to the body with remembrance of out-of-body experiences.

The healing sleep may also be used by patients for a range of healing experiences of which they are conscious. They can visit a special place, which is usually where they feel very happy.

They may also receive unique symbols or images, gain insights, receive information, have significant unions or reunions.

PATIENTS' OWN SOURCE OF GUIDANCE AND WISDOM

Patients always bring back something from a relaxation state that they need time to discuss, and to find their own interpretations and explanations for. This offers the healer an opportunity to point out how patients have accessed their own rich sources of guidance and wisdom. In all cases the healer is soul-centred, knowing that each patient has their own answer within.

To offer an interpretation of the patient's images or any other experiential material would be highly disempowering and against the ethos of the soul-based approach. But images and visions do play an important part in the healing process of many patients, as we shall see in the next chapter.

12

Sacred Tools: Visioning

Guided visualizations have been found to be effective in creating scenarios for mental relaxation, accessing inner guidance and in self-healing, and its use as a healing tool is already well documented. (For example, you will find examples of visualization exercises in Chapter 9 of *Your Healing Power*). In visualization the mind's power of imagination is used to create the image. The healer's role is to match the appropriate visualization experience to the patient's story.

The difference between imagining/visualizing and visioning is in where the image originates. In visioning, the image is first created by *soul*, then transmitted by mind as a visual experience.

An experience common to most indigenous healers is known as seeking a vision. The healer prays to be given a vision that will offer healing. This may also take the form of guidance, teaching or illustrate the solution to a problem. This is a powerful way of accessing soul guidance where the 'answer' to the prayer is presented as one or more images. The vision will be unique to the 'patient' and will generally have meaning for them only.

Visions have always been acknowledged by religions as having a divine origin and people who have them have been singled out as different or special. However, in practice and given the right circumstances, anyone is capable of having a vision.

Spiritual Healing harnesses our ability to gain access to the voice of soul in this way as a sacred tool of healing so that the 'external' healer becomes the 'internal' healer.

While many healers receive images related to the patient, it can be disempowering and unnecessary to offer your own material. Within Spiritual Healing the focus is on restoring the patient's ability to access their own guidance, teaching and solutions.

THE HEALING VISION

In the following stories, we show how, when the patient is given the right conditions, their innate ability to receive a visual message is used by soul to facilitate their healing.

In the first case, the relationship with the patient was well established and she was easily able to fall into a healing sleep during her sessions. In this deeply relaxed state, the patient accessed her own inner guidance in the form of a vision, which initiated many levels of healing.

Amelia, aged 54, was taking medication for depression. But she was still unable to sleep at night and her digestive problems continued. Her GP referred her for healing.

Amelia said she was grateful for the love and support provided by her two married daughters following the death of her husband five years previously. She had tried to make a new life for herself but was now very anxious about doing the right thing. A year ago she had met a man at her Spanish evening class. Their relationship had developed quickly. He had proposed marriage and a new life in Spain. Thrilled, she shared her news with her daughters. Their reaction shocked and hurt her. How could she think about leaving them after all they had done for her? Amelia was in a state of torment.

The first healing session helped her to relax. After the third session she was able to sleep through the night and after the sixth session her digestive disorder was beginning to ease. During one particular session, Amelia quickly slipped into a healing sleep as healing energy was directed to her heart, solar plexus and throat centres.

On awakening, Amelia told how she had been flying. The joy of flying shone in her eyes. 'I was on the back of this huge eagle. I could feel the feathers. I was holding on to the feathers. It was so fantastic – so high, so free, so much space. I felt wonderful. If only I could feel like that again.'

Amelia needed reassurance that she would find the answer to her dilemma. She continued her weekly healing sessions. Three weeks later, in her deeply relaxed state, she found herself flying again. This time she awoke announcing that she had got her answer. She told of her delight at flying again, but this time she had been aware of another eagle flying beside her. Looking across she saw her husband flying alongside her. He blew her a kiss.

'It was so beautiful. I'm going to Spain with Arthur and I've got my darling husband's blessing!'

The next story describes how the patient is invited to focus on the area of distress in her body, using her hands to reinforce the focus, and to see if an image comes into her vision, which will throw light on the presenting condition.

Margot had been experiencing problems with her digestion for a number of years. Medication had helped manage the distressing condition, but Margot wanted to be free of the pain. She was sure there was something else she could do and decided to try healing.

Margot was helped to relax her body and mind. She was asked to focus her awareness on the area of pain in her stomach and to allow an image to present itself. Margot placed her hands over her solar plexus.

Into her mind came the image of a large yellow disc. Then she saw a male figure, stripped to the waist, with his back to her. As she watched, she saw him pick up a large hammer and hit the yellow disc, which began to split into numerous small cracks. The pain increased. With each blow the disc continued to crack.

Then, as the figure once again raised the hammer above his head and took aim, Margot shouted out loud, 'Oh, no you don't, that's enough. Stop it!' The figure dropped the hammer and was gone. Margot cried with relief as she found her stomach pain easing. During the visioning, healing energy was directed to the solar plexus and brow centres. Over

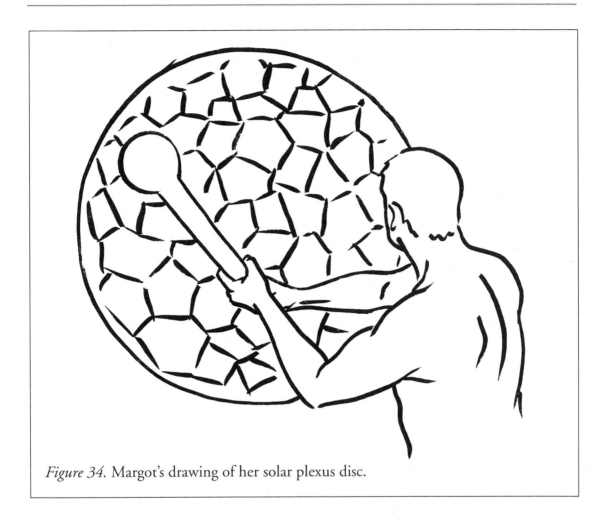

Figure 34. Margot's drawing of her solar plexus disc.

the course of the healing, the cracks in her solar plexus disc were healed until Margot saw that it was beautiful, shiny, golden and whole and she had become completely free of pain.

Margot had recognized the figure in her vision. This helped her to understand and begin healing the impact of a very unhappy marriage.

Margot's vision showed her the key to her stomach pain. Her body had been relaying her soul message, but she needed help to understand the cause of the pain. Soul found a way of empowering her by showing her the situation and that it was in her hands to bring about change.

Philip's story describes how the patient may receive a symbolic vision showing what is happening during the healing.

Philip had a history of respiratory illness related to many years of working in an unhealthy environment. The relaxation induced by the healing helped make breathing easier.

One day Philip asked if there was anything he could do to help himself. I suggested that he could explore visioning. Perhaps he would find a way of building on the healing sessions.

Philip closed his eyes, relaxed in the chair and was gently guided to

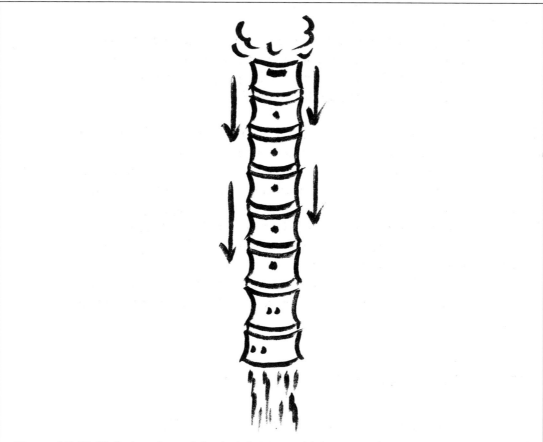

Figure 35. Philip's drawing of the bamboo recorder.

connect with his chest. Healing energy was directed to the throat, heart and solar plexus centres and the channel connecting them.

Meanwhile, he was invited to allow an image to come to him. He described what looked like a piece of bamboo. As he watched it became a recorder. 'I used to play the recorder when I was a schoolboy. I couldn't play one now though,' he joked.

The sadness he felt about his condition could be sensed in his heart centre as it called for more healing energy. Philip was encouraged to focus on the image of the recorder. As he watched, he saw himself blowing into the mouthpiece and was amazed at the 'gunge' he saw pouring out at the bottom. He was encouraged to hold his vision for as long as he felt comfortable. After a few minutes, tears of relief flowed as he felt his breathing become a little easier.

Despite being virtually crippled with this industrial disease, Philip had accessed a way of easing the distress of his condition. He would practise visualizing himself blowing the recorder. He laughed, 'Well, I'm going home to tell my wife I'm taking up the recorder!'

Here again, healing was occurring on many levels, showing the beauty and love with which soul is able to present the healing experience.

A fascinating aspect of visioning in Spiritual Healing (in contrast with visualization) is the way in which it bypasses mind conditioning – the soul message is always delivered intact. We emphasize that the appropriate conditions of attunement and Sacred Mindfulness have to be established by the healer so that the patient and the atmosphere can be held energetically to support the arrival of the soul material.

With this in mind, the next Action Point is designed to give you and a partner the opportunity to experience accessing a healing vision and working with it.

ACTION POINT 42 Visioning to Heal a Condition

Developmental tool – working with the creative facility of mind to produce and/or receive symbolic representation of the energetic pattern of a condition.

This exercise may also be used as a self-healing activity to promote relationship with a condition and suggest action to be taken.

You and your partner will need to achieve a state of attunement together that is conducive to healing. Refer to the section on Attunement of Self *in Chapter 6. Once you have both attuned together, you should lie on a healing couch or sit on a chair with your partner sitting close by. Your partner should read out the rest of the instructions for the exercise.*

- Close your eyes and go within. Focus on your breath and your breathing. See yourself taking in all the energy you are needing at this time and let go on the out-breath.

- Allow yourself to become calm and feel yourself becoming more relaxed with every out-breath, letting go against the couch (in the chair) and against the pillow.

- Without grasping at it, let a condition come to mind that you would like to work with. Let this condition be present without directing any energy to it, by thinking about it or by dwelling on it.

- If you experience the condition in your body, place your hands there. Notice if your hands seem to want to go somewhere else on your body. Let them find where they want to rest.

- Your breathing will show you if you can be present in a relaxed way with this condition, with any pain/discomfort, and with any thoughts or feelings that may arise. Allow your breathing to help you stay calm and relaxed.

- Invite an image to come now that relates to the condition in some way. You may want to ask, 'What do I need to know?' or, 'Show me what I need to see'.

- Staying calm and relaxed allow the image to appear. It may take a few moments.

- Spend time with the image and try not to grasp at it. Remember your breathing. Be the observer without needing to understand the image or to work it out at this stage.

- Notice any details. Quietly describe what you are seeing.

- Spend as long as feels comfortable with the image. It will signal when it is time to let go by gradually fading.

- Do not try to hold on to the image. Let it slip away. You can help it with your out-breath.

- Give thanks and bring your attention back to your breath and your breathing. With every in-breath feel yourself returning gently to a normal wakened state. With every out-breath let go of the visioning.

- Gradually become aware of your body lying on the couch (sitting in the chair). Use your breathing to help you connect fully with your physical body and your surroundings.

- Open your eyes and spend a few minutes relating to your surroundings.

- When you feel ready, discuss your experience with your partner. Work with your partner to make sense of the image.

- As a result of your experience is there anything you need to do or say? Share this with your partner.

- You may want to draw/illustrate your image to record the healing experience and/or to continue working with the image and its unique message.

As you will note from this Action Point, it may be very helpful for the patient to engage their creativity to record their experience in some way. The image or object will then serve as a focus for further work with their soul message.

The stories of so many patients have shown us that everyone has a vision of how life on Earth should be and that they are born with a vision in which they see their unique role in the creation of it. It is the image of their soul mission.

A person's reaction to life experience may cloud this vision or put them out of touch with it completely. Nevertheless it still exists. As the stories of Amelia,

Margot and Philip have illustrated, ill health may be the catalyst that impels them to reconnect with or access their vision. The essence of visioning in Spiritual Healing is to create the circumstances where they can do this.

13

Sacred Tools:
Intuitive Awareness

NATURAL HUMAN ABILITIES – PSYCHIC AND
INTUITIVE AWARENESS

Modern societies have a problem with intuition and all that has been termed 'psychic'. If they do exist, how can they be quantified and, if they cannot be quantified, do they exist? Some people wrestle with such questions while the rest of us supply a commonsense answer.

The detective character who acts on his hunches is loved by readers and TV audiences alike, but is a thorn in the side of his superiors. Men get upset when women act on a 'feeling' they have about something. People feel impelled to cancel a holiday trip without knowing why, only later to be shown how their intuition was correct. We have all walked into an empty room and felt an atmosphere 'you could cut with a knife' – we knew something was going on in there, such as a row. Have you ever turned round for no reason to find someone watching you intently?

These awarenesses are a normal, everyday occurrence and a natural ability we all possess. This function of the brow centre, and the brain's interpretation of it, are part of our survival equipment. What a shame, then, that it is not embraced as an essential part of human development and something that should feature in every child's education (recall William Wordsworth's gift of inner vision in Chapter 7). Instead, the general suppression, denial and fear of both psychic and intuitive awareness is a great loss to the community. This has come about because of the problem we mentioned earlier, with its historical echoes of suppression by the Christian church and, later, the ridicule of certain scientific circles.

In some people, their psychic and/or intuitive awareness is so highly developed that they have a job to convince others that their perceptions are a valid part of their experience and not some form of mental ill health. Consequently, they may prefer to just keep quiet about it. Yet a musician or a mathematician who shows great ability is accepted as a 'genius' or 'prodigy'.

If you walked into a cloud of radioactive air you would not know it and you would suffer the consequences of your ignorance. But someone with a Geiger counter would have registered the radioactivity. The person with a well-developed psychic or intuitive awareness is like this – she has a means of detection, which is her excellent ability to co-ordinate subtle energetic information, supplied by her brow centre, with her brain's facility to make sense of it. Without this developed awareness, we pass by regardless.

THE DIFFERENCE BETWEEN PSYCHIC AND INTUITIVE AWARENESS

Part of the general confusion about psychic ability and intuitive awareness is the assumption that they are the same thing. Healers use both and need to be fully aware of the difference between and the purposes of these two gifts of perception.

Psychic awareness

Psychic awareness is the natural human ability to sense subtle energetic phenomena, including clairvoyance and clairaudience. Think of this sixth sense to be as necessary as the other five.

Since subtle phenomena originate outside of the space/time frame (because they vibrate faster than the speed of light), some of them may be perceived as relating to future or past time. Hence some people have the ability known as 'precognition'.

The instances described earlier, such as sensing the atmosphere in an empty room and the ability to 'see' the subtle energy radiations of people, animals and plants (as we quoted in Wordsworth, for example), are typical psychic awarenesses that are patently useful to us. They are received by the brow centre and sent to the solar plexus for processing (by mind). But when a person is surrounded by the fear or denial of psychic awareness, mind will find ways to close down interpretation and eventually repress the ability. This is what has happened to many people in western societies.

So-called 'psychic' occurences are those that can only be detected through psychic awareness, hence they have been termed *occult* (hidden), with all the negative connotations that this word has accumulated.

Yet, for many, psychic ability is a route into healing. It should be accepted, validated and nurtured as a valuable gift.

Intuitive awareness

The brow also receives other subtle energetic information. Where psychic information is about *external* subtle energetic events, intuitive information is about internal events – information coming from a soul/spirtual level.

Soul directs the total healing process so that it is *intuitive* awareness, which is used as a sacred tool to maintain alignment with soul. This keeps us open to soul guidance.

The Action Points in this chapter encourage you to focus in this way so that you begin to sense when material is being presented by the soul. Think of intuitive awareness as the 'seventh sense', which many would prize as more valuable than the other six!

Psychic awareness has received much attention and has become the way of explaining intuitive awareness. Here, we make a plea for distinguishing between these two exceptional gifts of communication.

THE PURPOSE OF PRECOGNITION

An example of an unacknowledged gift to the community is the aspect of awareness known as as 'precognition'. Here, the person is shown details of an event, such as an accident or traumatic happening, which has yet to take place, and wonders what to do about it. The reactions of others tend to range from incredulity or indifference to feeling sorry for the person.

We have known many people who felt their lives were blighted by precognition experiences because they did not know how to deal with them and did not know where to go for help and understanding. They also did not know if the experience was at a psychic or intuitive level.

If a person feels that precognition is an unwelcome *psychic* ability, they can move it to the level of loving service by asking soul to indicate how the material can be used to benefit others. This may be done by entering a meditative state, after making the request, and waiting patiently for soul's response. In our experience, precognition is soul's message saying, 'Get ready, you can help, either literally or by sending out love and healing to the situation. It is not a pressure on you to prevent it happening unless you are actually in a position to do this'.

LINKING WITH INTUITIVE AWARENESS

As we saw in Chapter 4, many indigenous peoples still make use of the faculty of intuitive awareness both to enrich everyday life and to ensure the proper development of the healer or shaman. Because the soul-based approach depends on your ability to listen to soul, the majority of the Action Points in this book will develop your intuitive awareness and your capacity to make use of your awareness.

The first place that we hear soul is at a subtle level in the brow centre. The message then moves to the heart, then to the solar plexus, where it is checked out by mind and is immediately redirected to the heart. The movement of the soul message to the heart allows you to identify the loving aspect of the material – which distinguishes it from psychic information.

Your open-heartedness and an open mind to the voice of soul is what we have encouraged you to practise. From the moment you feel, 'I would like to help', first ask yourself why this is and then ask for soul guidance. Sit quietly, relax and go into your heart centre. Wait patiently for your heart's answer.

Try to be aware (beware) of the ego's need to feel good, to feel wanted, for that pat on the back, for grateful thanks, for admiration. These self-centred needs can, unfortunately, stand in the way of intuitive awareness and, thus, soul guidance.

In Spiritual Healing, the healer is encouraged to return to the question of motivation again and again. And this has relevance for every time you go to do healing, not simply for the beginner. Questioning your motivation keeps the channel pure and also avoids burnout. Your answers will point out your motivation for wanting to help.

If you are satisfied with your inner answer, you are ready to tune in to your inner awareness. The next time you are confronted with a situation where you feel you could offer help, ask yourself, 'What do my hands want to do?' Focus on them, realizing their link with the heart centre. Your question is again addressed to this link where you are asking the heart for guidance. Notice what happens.

ARE YOU A HEALER?

As we discussed in Chapter 9, Sacred Mind – Sacred Feeling, the programmed mind may block inner guidance so that some people are presented instead with a confusing mixture of doubts and queries. Many people ask us, 'Do you think I'm a healer?' or 'Could you teach me how to heal?' Others say, 'I've been told I'm a healer' or 'So and so says I should heal, what do you think?'

Our first reaction is to get them to talk about it. How do they feel when someone else tells them who they are or what they should be doing? Together we explore how they feel in their heart about being able to help another. On their life path, have they been drawn to healing in some other way or even reluctantly? These important issues, and their implications, need time and sensitivity to be addressed. This allows potential healers to gain some insight into how and how not to talk to their patients and into how patients may be disempowered.

Insight opens up the lines of communication between our intuition and our mind and is very often the result of linking with soul guidance. A healer is a gift to the community, so it is important for them to develop the heart centre energy of compassion through learning how to understand others. Intuition will guide them in how best to do this.

CREATING GROUP ENERGY

For most people, the next step is to explore being part of a group and experiencing group energies. We use the following Action Point to link group members in love. It is a simple but profound way of attunement. Use it to start any piece of work with a friend/partner or with a group. Group facilitators will be able to monitor, or can learn how to monitor, individual experiencing and the management of energy.

ACTION POINT 43 Linking Together To Begin Work

Developmental tool – exploring awareness of the heart centre and giving/receiving this energy within the context of a group.

- The group or partnership should sit together quietly. Relax the body, using the breath to bring calm, then breathe normally.

- Light a candle and dedicate the light to the group and your work together.

- Ask for protection and the guidance of soul.

- See the light of the candle as the light of the soul and breathe it into the heart centre. This opens up the heart centre.

- Now pass the energy in your heart centre to the person on your left until you are all linked together in common purpose. Intuitively, you may have to wait to gather your heart energy and, in the waiting, you gain insight into the condition of your heart centre. This core of the ceremony thus has four parts – waiting, gathering the energy, intuitively sensing the state of your heart centre, and sending the energy on.

- This is a moment for any personal prayers that group members might like to say aloud. Finally, give thanks for the opportunity to work together and offer the work to the Source.

This ceremony of 'passing the love round' creates a powerful group energy, even with one other person, which is inherently healing in nature and beneficial in effect. It sends a signal to the intuitive side that this is a safe place, where people can experience individual gifts and where individual gifts will be validated.

It provides the opportunity for expressing gratitude. When something is offered or given, gratitude has the effect on a subtle level of actually helping the circulation of this energy.

Gratitude acknowledges soul and affirms your trust in life, the Source and your own self.

The simplicity of the ceremony demonstrates how love is always available. Within the support of the group, each person is able to experience giving and receiving love, which is what healing is all about. In this way, you begin to work with the sacred cycle of love.

INTUITIVE AWARENESS IN ACTION

Once you have created your unique group or partnership energy, you are ready to put your inner guidance to work and ready to be directed from the heart. We use the next Action Point with groups at an early stage in training. The exercise helps people to find out if they *do* have innate ability as a healer and if they can tap into their own inner guidance to use it. You should try to work with at least two other people.

ACTION POINT 44 Using Intuitive Awareness (I)

Developmental tool – responding to intuitive impulses received by the heart and followed with the hands.

Divide into pairs. In a group of three, one person acts as an observer, experiencing with the heart and staying open to individual promptings to offer later.

- Have your partner lie on a healing couch or sit on a chair. Stand at the foot of the couch or just opposite your seated partner.

- Put your mind in your heart centre and be aware of its links with your two palm centres. Wait until you feel this connection.

- Spend a few moments being aware of your partner and their energy field. Notice any impressions/sensations.

- Ask yourself, 'Where do my hands want to go?'

- Do not wait for a mental reply, but straight away let your hands be guided to move towards your partner's body or energy field. If you feel your hands want to work on the physical, do not touch your partner, but keep your palms about 5 to 10cm away from your partner's body.

- Hold them over the area and see what you sense.

- If you feel you need to go to a second or third place, move slowly in each case.

- Your hands will tell you when you have done all you can by coming to a stop. Move your hands slowly away from your partner and step away from the couch or chair.

- Mentally thank your partner.

- Compare notes. Discuss your experience with your partner. What do they have to say about the areas your hands visited? Change over. Compare notes again. In each case assess how the hand work matched the partner's story. In a group of three, make sure to include the observer's comments.

- Repeat the procedure with a new partner. In a group of three, each person should have the chance to take each role. Again, compare notes, assessing how the hand work matched the partner's story.

- If you have been working with a group, meet again to discuss your experiences. Try to sum up what you all feel you have learned together.

Here are some examples of healing awareness in our group sessions. In each case, no information was given to members before the sensing.

> Dieter went immediately to the person's right forearm and from there to the lower left leg and ankle. The story was that the person had been in a skiing accident some three years before and had broken his right arm and left leg and ankle.
>
> Maria went to a place on the body where a woman had had major surgery.
>
> In Roberto's case, his hands wanted to move all over the person's body. He trusted his intuition and later learned that the person suffered from psoriasis over a large part of his body.
>
> Kuniko had to trust her intuitive awareness when her hands stopped quite a way from her partner's body. This lady was still grieving over the death of her dog and Kuniko's hands needed to work on the emotional, rather than the physical level.

In the examples above, the partner's story matches the healer's hand awareness. But many of these awarenesses could have been perceived psychically. However, when awareness is *intuitive*, soul adds the heart qualities of unconditional love and compassion, deeper insights into causes and guidance about treatment. Thus, there is no right or wrong, good or bad in this work, only practice, progress and building on your experience. So, if your sensing experience is not corroborated by your partner/patient, make a note of it as part of your own database. Sooner or later you will receive your own answers and insights.

Now try out the next Action Point. You should know nothing about your 'patient'. This time we have a different approach.

ACTION POINT 45 Using Intuitive Awareness (2)

Developmental tool – monitoring intuitive impulses; practising communicating in a sacred manner.

Divide up into groups of three – a healer, a patient, an observer.

- Sit together, relax and breathe into the heart centre. Try to keep your focus here.

- Work the same way as before. This time, in addition, ponder these questions:

  - **Healer** What is this soul 'saying' to me during this exercise?

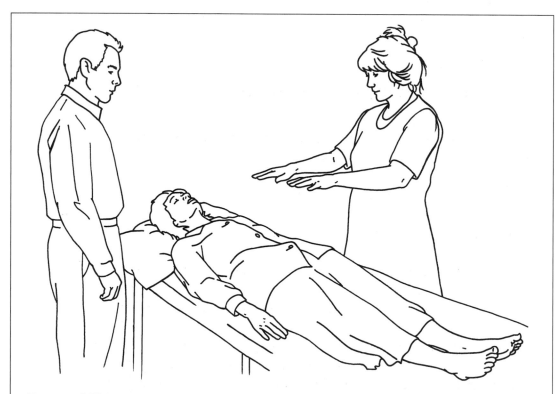

Figure 36. Using intuitive awareness. The healer is seeing where her hands want to go in the patient's field. The observer is also sensing intuitively.

- **Observer** What is the healer 'saying' to the patient?

- **Patient** What do I find myself 'saying' to the healer?

- Compare notes together. Change round so that each person has a chance to experience each role.

- If you have been working with a group, meet again to discuss your experiences. What happens when you focus on what soul is 'saying'? This exercise is about sharing feelings, intuition and hunches, not what you *think* the patient is saying or signalling. Try to sum up what you all feel you have learned together.

Just as you opened your piece of work with a ceremony, close it in a similar way, as described below, so that you are reminded about the sacred cycle of the work.

ACTION POINT 46 Closing the Work Session

Developmental tool – promoting responsibility for energetic signalling of completion of work.

- Sit together again. You may wish to link hands.

- Give thanks for the work and what you have learned.

- Blow out the dedicated light of the candle by asking a group member to 'send the light out'. This could be sent to a person, an animal, a place or situation – whatever comes intuitively to mind is right for that moment.

If, after the close of your work, you are going to travel or go to a different energetic environment, you should now carry out the Clearing, Centre Regulation and Protection exercises in Chapter 5, A Way of Being (Action Points 8, 9 and 10).

INTUITIVE AWARENESS – A GIFT TO YOUR PATIENT

Well, was your intuitive awareness working and did you know where your palm centres needed to go? After working with Action Points 39 and 40, review the whole session in private to see if your basic queries about yourself and healing have been answered.

We only introduce the healing scans to trainees when they and we are satisfied that they intuitively know where their hands 'want to go' and that this matches the stories of their trainee partners or volunteer patients. This means that they are in touch with their soul guidance and will not base their healing practice on a set procedure, such as a healing scan or their interpretation of subtle energetic information alone. The procedure is not the healing, neither is the carrying out of the procedure. The healing is using the procedure with heart – soul working with and for soul.

Along with conscious breathing, conscious relaxation and visioning, your intuitive awareness is a gift to your patient and a sacred tool of healing.

SELF-HEALING

If you consider that this section applies to you, we are glad that you do not see yourself as separate from your patients and acknowledge that you too may need help sometimes.

We have clearly indicated throughout which Action Points are appropriate for self-healing. Just like working with someone else, it is very much a question of soul-guidance and the intuitive way. When looking at yourself, it is necessary to be as objective as possible. Your Sacred Mindfulness practice will help you to gain an objective view of yourself.

Augment the self-healing potential of an Action Point by addressing your presenting condition. When you have calmed yourself and reached a state of harmony by using the breathing and relaxation exercises you have practised, you are ready to offer yourself up to intuitive guidance. If it is a physical condition that you are experiencing, work with your body. Ask, 'What do I need to know about this condition?' Allow it to speak to you. Whether it is an organ, a system, a pain or sensation, move in close with your awareness and ask for guidance. Wait patiently for your answer.

Similarly, if you are suffering emotional or mental distress, accept your experience and move in close to it. Be present with it. What does it want to say to you? Have you considered that it is possible to experience pain without suffering? Ask the condition to show you how this may be possible.

When you feel you have done all you can to be intimate with your body and its systems, ask for soul-guidance on how you can help yourself. Now where do your hands need to go?

A healer with many years' experience told us that she always put herself 'top of the list', in terms of healing help. 'People who think I'm self-centred don't understand,' she said. 'After all, if I get ill I can't help them, can I?'

Are you 'top of the list' or the last to receive consideration? Self-healing is about Oneness not self-centredness. When you take time to practise this form of the Sacred Meeting, you enhance the energy field, which you later offer your patients.

14

The Sacred Meeting

On the door to our therapy room hangs a piece of calligraphy, a present from a Japanese female artist. Over the years many patients have passed through the doorway without noticing this beautifully painted ideogram. Then sometimes things like this happen:

One day Leroy arrived for his first healing session. He had a number of conditions related to his long-standing diabetes. On entering the healing room Leroy paused, looked at the calligraphy and said, 'That is so beautiful, tell me, what does it mean?'

'It's Japanese for "light",' I explained.

With a huge grin Leroy went on into the healing room. 'This way to the light!', he roared.

How right he is, I thought.

Since Leroy's first visit we have noticed an interesting phenomenon. When patients enter or leave the healing room and comment on the calligraphy, significant progress has been made in their healing.

If you have practised all the Action Points so far, you will have gone a long way to creating a clear hollow bone, your channel for the Light. You will also have begun to notice the effect that light (healing energy) is having on your-

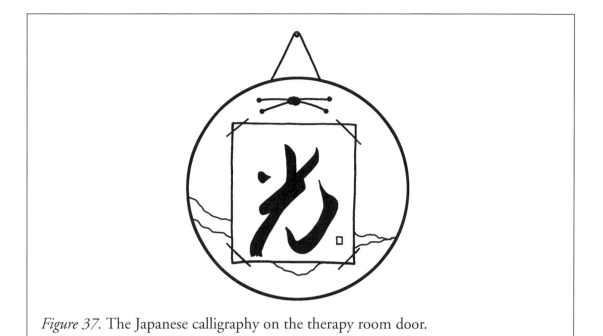

Figure 37. The Japanese calligraphy on the therapy room door.

self as well as your environment. Now you are ready to work with the light of soul, you will see in this chapter how the relevant Action Points have brought you safely to the healing session. Everything you have made a part of you will be called upon when you begin the practice of Spiritual Healing. This is what you will be offering your patients.

In a sense there have already been sacred meetings between your personality and your soul, and between yourself and a partner or group. These meetings have prepared you for the Sacred Meeting you knew intuitively you wanted to have – the encounter with another soul who has asked for your help.

PRELIMINARIES

Before inviting your patients into the sacred space you have created, you need to have also brought yourself into a state of attunement with the Source and with your soul (see Chapter 6, Preparing Sacred Space). The second preliminary is to check the furniture – the chairs and healing couch, check that the linen, pillows and blanket for the couch are clean, check your music, if you use it, check that there is water to drink and that there are tissues available. Check that you are relaxed and aware.

THE HEALING SESSION

Energetic activity, in a healing sense, begins as soon as the patient enters the therapy room. Seated opposite you, they need time to adjust to their new energetic environment. During this time you are listening attentively, as they express aspects of their journey and what they are seeking healing for. This exposes these aspects to the light. You are listening in a soul-centred way, not needing to give advice and knowing that the patient has their own answer. In the healing environment of the sacred space, whatever is requested attracts energy to it. At the same time, you are sensing their energy field and beginning to attune to them.

Ask whether they have had healing before and explain what you are going to do. Offer them couch or chair healing. Ask them whether they can be touched because your signal for the beginning and end of the healing procedure will be to touch them lightly on the shoulders or ankles. If they cannot be touched you will need to use a different signal. The only items of clothing the patient will need to remove would be an outer coat and footwear.

We recommend working on the healing couch wherever possible, with access to all sides of it. It is far easier to access the patient's body and they have the chance to fully relax, or to go into the healing sleep (see Chapter 11, Sacred Tools: Breathing and Relaxation) without worrying about falling off a chair. If you do not have access to all sides of the couch, adapt your body position accordingly.

Action Point 47, below, deals with the procedure on the couch. This will be followed by Action Point 48, the chair procedure. You will need to become familiar with both procedures.

ACTION POINT 47 The Healing Procedure – Patient on the Couch

Celebrating your learning by bringing it all together for the purpose of Spiritual Healing.

You will need to record this Action Point or get a third person to read it to you. To avoid confusion, we will call your partner 'the patient'. Take your time and, while you are learning, stop at the end of scans if you need to. You are ready to work with a patient when you have internalized the structure of the healing procedure and are in tune with its rhythm.

Beginning the procedure, relaxing the patient

The patient lies on the couch and is made comfortable, with no arms or legs crossed, and with no link between the hands. A pillow should support the neck and, if there is back discomfort, the patient's legs should be raised at the knees and supported with another pillow. Ask if they would like a blanket to cover them.

The patient should be lying on their back at all times.

Check that you are relaxed and aware. If you have not been guided already, stand a few paces away from the couch while you check whether you need to start at the patient's shoulders or ankles.

Most procedures start at the shoulders. Tell your patient where you will be starting and what your signal will be to begin and end the healing procedure. Unless the patient objects, this will be a light touch on the shoulders. Step up to the couch and lightly put your hands on the patient. While you are doing this, mentally thank the patient and ask for permission to work with them. This sends a signal of acknowledgement to the soul (Figure 38).

Now talk them through a basic breathing and relaxation exercise (such as Action Point 38), keeping your hands on the shoulders. Give positive comments to signal that you see what they are achieving. Many patients find it difficult to relax, especially if it is their first experience of healing, and may need reassurance. When you feel the patient is relaxed and ready, move into position to carry out the energy centre scan.

(If you are intuitively impressed to start at the ankles, step up to the end of the couch and lightly put your hands there. Make sure that your patient

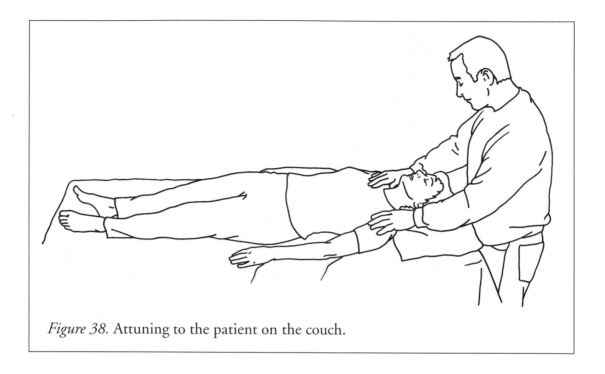

Figure 38. Attuning to the patient on the couch.

knows that this is your signal to start and end the healing. Follow the procedure for the shoulders. Then step up to the other end of the couch for the energy centre scan).

The energy centre scan

The scans prepare the system for healing. They also introduce the healer's energy to the patient's system. For the purpose of the Action Point, we will assume that you are standing on the left side of the patient.

Stand near the patient's head, with your left arm relaxed by your side and your right arm outstretched, to sense the crown centre energy channel of the patient's aura. Move your right hand to follow the track of the energy channel through the aura towards the crown centre (Figure 39).

Once you feel a change in the activity in your hand (which suggests that it is no longer scanning), put your left palm opposite your patient's brow centre, at the etheric level (about 10 to 15cm from the body). The first scan is at this etheric level and should be carried out at this level until you reach

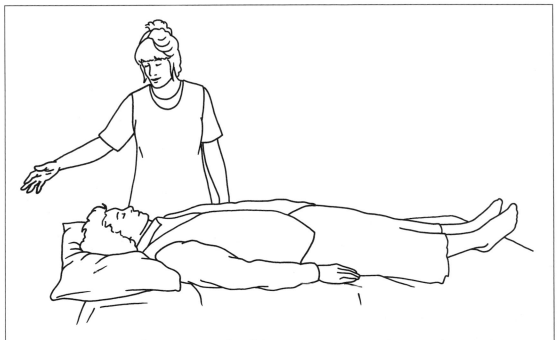

Figure 39. Sensing the energy track of the crown centre, patient on the couch.

the base. When you feel you have completed the scan of the brow, move your left palm to the throat and follow with the right to the brow. You will sense that the left hand is scanning the centre, while your right hand follows to channel the healing. In this way you are always in a position to compare the energy of two centres. Let your hands be guided to decide how long they need to remain at each centre. You should notice a change in sensation, which coincides with the movement from one centre to the next.

As you move from centre to centre, be aware that you are also scanning and working with the central channel, linked to each centre, in the same way.

Make a mental note of your sensations and impressions later to build up your database (Figure 40).

Move your left palm to the heart and follow with the right to the throat.

Move your left palm to the solar plexus and follow with the right to the heart.

Move your left palm to the sacral and follow with the right to the solar plexus.

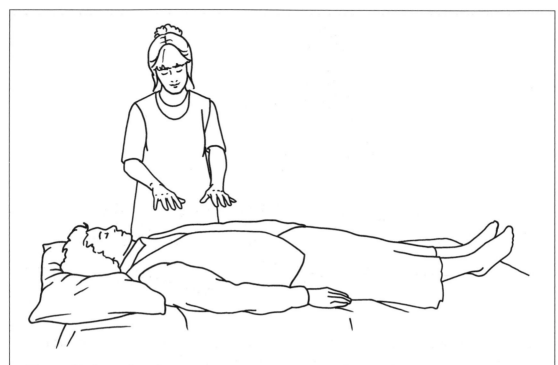

Figure 40. Scanning the energy centres, patient on the couch. The healer is scanning the heart and solar plexus.

Move your left palm to the base and follow with the right to the sacral. Move the left from the base along the energy track within the aura and follow with the right to the base. Move the right hand along the energy track of the base into the aura. Hold the left hand opposite the energy track of the base centre. A final sensing will reveal whether the central channel is balanced or calling for more energy (Figure 41).

All your movements should be slow, gentle and purposeful.

Five links anchor the subtle bodies to the physical

Now move to work with the five energy centre links (see Chapter 8, Seven Sacred Steps). With these links, the healer reunites the subtle bodies with the physical.

With the first link the physical is linked with the soul.

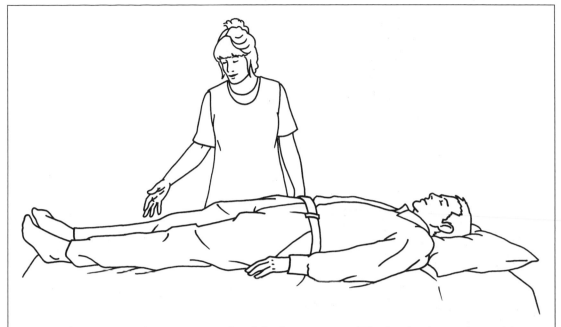

Figure 41. Sensing the energy track of the base centre. The healer is sensing with the right palm when working from the patient's right hand.

The emotional 'body' is anchored in the physical via the sacral centre. When the link is complete it is sensed in the throat centre.

The mental 'body' is anchored in the physical via the solar plexus centre. The completed link is sensed in the brow centre.

The soul is anchored in the physical via the heart centre (as in the first linking). Then the linking has to be sensed as the energy moves up from the heart to the crown and then down the central channel, so that the base, heart and crown are linked.

Scanning the five energy centre links

Hold the left palm opposite the base, with the right opposite the heart. Sense the energetic activity bringing the link to a state of balance.

Move the left palm to the sacral and the right to the throat. Proceed as before.

Move the left palm to the solar plexus and the right to the brow. Proceed as before.

Move the left palm to the heart and the right to the crown. Proceed as before.

Move the left palm to the base and keep the right at the crown. Proceed as before.

Now return to the feet to check the balance of the polarities (as in Action Point 18). Observe the patient while you are getting a sense of balance in the patient's field.

The skeletal energy circuit scan

Having completed the scanning and healing of the centres, at an etheric level, proceed with scanning and healing the energy circuits associated with the skeleton. This is your healing intention.

Hold the hands near the top of the head (about 5 to 10cm from the body). Move one hand slowly over the top of the head and across the face to locate where the spine joins the base of the skull. Move your leading (left) hand slowly over the spine until your hand is opposite its base in the coccyx, keeping your right hand opposite the base of the skull. Sense the energy between your two palms. Slowly bring your right hand down the spine to meet the left at the base.

Remember, the procedure in the skeletal circuit scan is in three parts: your leading hand is scanning and clearing the energy between two 'points'; your two palms hold and sense the balance between the two points; your following hand brings in the new healing energy. Be aware of any resistance to the movement of your hands. In this case, pause and wait for the energy to move your hands.

Remove your hands from opposite the base of the spine to work back at the head and to move down one side of the body (moving with the polarity). If it is the right side, then this is your leading hand. Starting at the head, move slowly down the right side of the face, over the cheek-bones and jaw, to the base of the neck. Follow with the left hand. Move your right hand slowly to the right shoulder and follow with the left. Move your right hand to the elbow and follow with the left. Move your right hand to the wrist and follow with the left. Move your right hand carefully over the fingers and follow with the left. Move your right hand gently out into the aura and follow with the left.

Return to the right shoulder and move your right hand down over the ribs to the right hip. Follow with the left.

Move both hands to be opposite the base of the spine and move the right across to the patient's right hip. Follow with the left. Move the right hand to the right knee and follow with the left, taking time with the long bones such as the thigh. Move the right hand to the ankle and follow with the left. Move the right hand out across the foot and toes. Follow with the left. Move your right hand out into the aura and follow with the left.

Repeat the procedure down the left side of the patient's body, starting at the left side of the head and finishing in the aura by the left foot, as before.

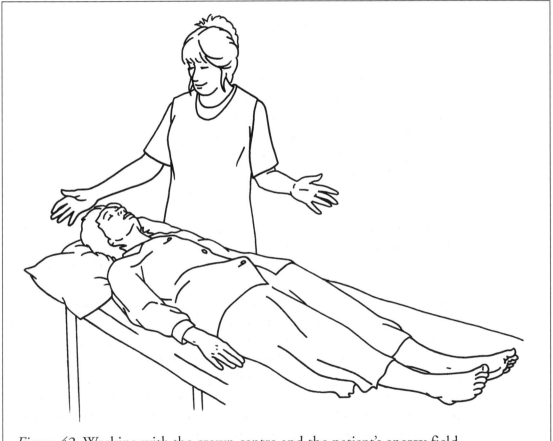

Figure 42. Working with the crown centre and the patient's energy field, patient on couch.

Check the balance of the skeletal energy circuits by holding the palms opposite the soles of the feet, as in Action Point 28. Observe the patient while you are getting a sense of balance and experiencing the condition of the skeleton.

This completes the first part of the healing procedure in which the energy scans have allowed the patient's system to open up and present you with an energetic diagnosis.

Working at a deeper level

The healing now moves to the second, consolidating part of the procedure, which is a deeper level of work. Here, as you intuitively work with the energetic diagnosis, you are effectively asking your hands, 'Where do you need to go now?'

Go back to where you feel you need to, based on the information that your hands have given you. This could be either to an energy centre, the skeletal circuit or somewhere on the physical. Work in that order, treating the centres first.

In the case of a centre, move to where in the energy field your hands need to go – is it still at an etheric level or has it moved to the emotional or mental? (Recall Action Point 25, when you sensed the location of an energy centre and its activity level.) In each case, wait for a change of sensation in your palms, which signals that healing has been given.

After completing this phase of the work, see if your intuition is still directing you somewhere. It might be to the feet, to do some more balancing, or to the crown centre. Here, one hand is held near the crown and the other is held out in the aura (Figure 42). If you feel intuitively that you need to go back to do some more healing, realize that this is a sign of your sensitivity to your patient's needs and soul direction. Each time you 'go back', the healing moves to a deeper level and to a different energetic mode.

Your patient may register awareness of the different levels of healing as this takes place. This could take the form of spontaneous facial and/or body movements and/or emotional release. There is no need to stop the healing procedure when a patient cries. Be reassuring without blocking the flow of the release. A gentle, 'Are you all right?', will signal that you are there and that you have noted their distress.

After each phase, return to the feet to check the balance of the patient. You may be called back to this balancing position many times during the healing. This is because it draws more light down into the system and, as new energy flows in, the two subtle systems of polarity need readjustment to maintain overall balance. The return to the balancing position is how the healer 'fine-tunes' the system as the healing progresses.

Other work may be called for by the patient (at a soul level). For example, you may feel the need to draw a hand from the crown through the centres to the base, as if checking that there is no further call from them.

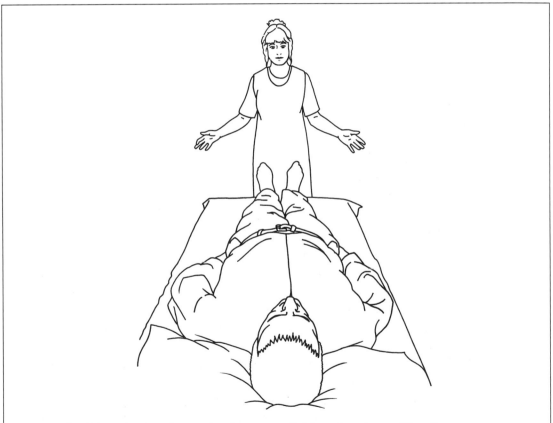

Figure 43. Directing to the patient's energy field at the close of healing, patient on couch.

Working at a deeper level occurs because the patient is needing it, and has been prepared for it by the earlier scans. This is why we encourage you to be fully aware intuitively and open to the promptings of the soul before you work with a patient.

Closing the healing procedure

The healing procedure ends when you find yourself at the patient's feet for the final time. Hold your hands out to direct to the aura. This is a good point at which to mentally give your thanks.

Give your patient the agreed signal that the healing is over. Gently talk them back to a normal waking state with your hands on their shoulders, just as they were when you talked them into the relaxation state at the beginning. Once they seem to be coming back, move to where they can see you. Encourage them to open their eyes, when they feel ready, and to spend a moment taking in where they are. Many patients feel the need to hold your hand at this point. Be ready for this, as it is an important signal that you are there for them and that they have returned safely to their body.

When you are sure that they are back (in their body), help them to sit up on the couch and to swing their legs round. Make sure no limbs are crossed. Check that their eyes are taking in their surroundings and assist them back to the meeting chair where the session began.

Before we describe the conclusion of the session, here is the healing procedure with the patient on the chair.

**ACTION POINT 48 The Healing Procedure –
Patient on the Chair**

Beginning the procedure, relaxing the patient

The patient sits on the chair and is made comfortable, with no arms or legs crossed, and with no link between the hands. The feet should be flat on the floor. Check that you are relaxed and aware.

If you have not been guided already, stand a few paces away from the chair

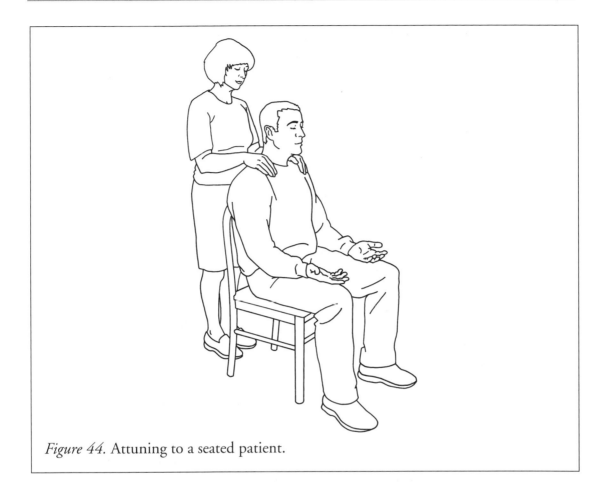

Figure 44. Attuning to a seated patient.

while you check whether you need to start at the patient's shoulders or ankles. Most procedures start at the shoulders. Tell your patient where you will be starting and what your signal will be to begin and end the healing procedure. Check whether they mind being touched. Step up to the chair and lightly put your hands on the patient. While you are doing this, mentally thank the patient and ask for permission to work with them. This sends a signal of acknowledgement to the soul.

Now talk them through a basic breathing and relaxation exercise, keeping your hands on the shoulders. Give positive comments to signal that you see what they are achieving. Many patients find it difficult to relax, especially if it is their first experience of healing, and may need reassurance. When you

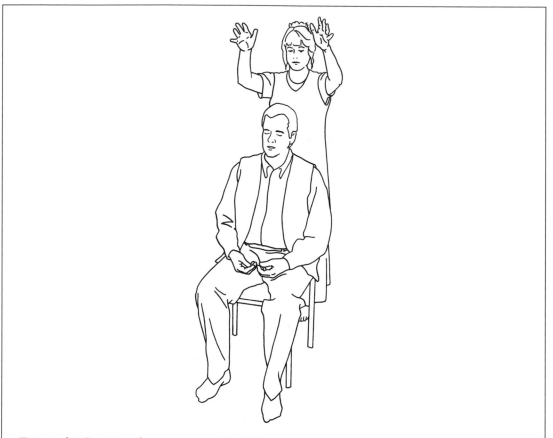

Figure 45. Sensing the energy track of the crown centre, patient on the chair.

feel the patient is relaxed and ready, move into position to carry out the energy centre scan.

(If you are intuitively impressed to start at the ankles, squat by your patient's feet and lightly put your hands there. Make sure your patient knows that this is your signal to start and end the healing. Follow the relaxation procedure, then proceed with the energy centre scan).

The energy centre scan

For the purpose of this Action Point, we will assume that you commence by standing behind the patient and that you then move to be on their left side.

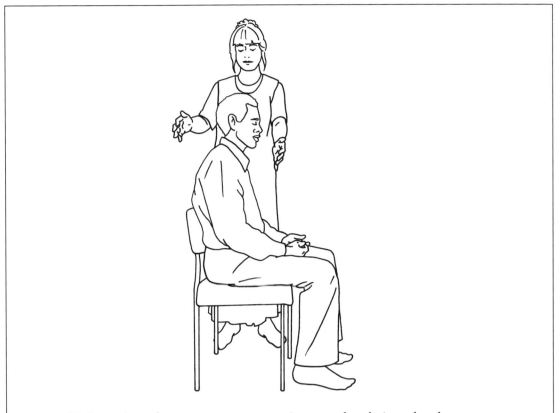

Figure 46. Scanning the energy centres, patient on the chair – the throat centre.

Stand with both arms outstretched above the patient's head to sense the crown centre energy channel of the patient's aura. Move your right hand to follow the track of the energy channel through the aura towards the crown centre. Once you feel a change in the activity in your right hand (which suggests that it is no longer scanning), gently bring your left hand so that your two hands are above the crown centre at the etheric level (about 10 to 15cm from the body), but separated by the width of the patent's head. The first scan is at this etheric level and should be carried out at this level until you reach the base.

Step to the left side of your patient. Gently move both palms opposite your patient's brow centre, with the right palm at the back of the head.

When you feel you have completed the scan of the brow, move both your palms to the throat centre, with the right at the back of the neck.

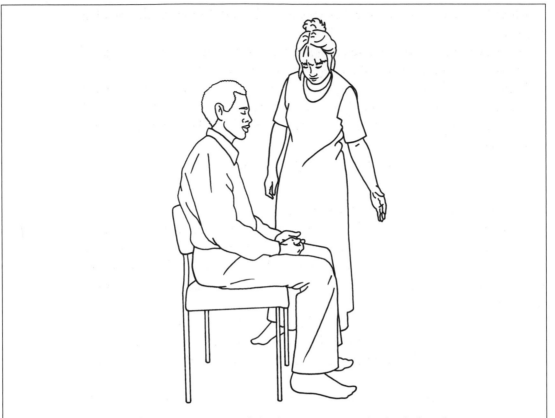

Figure 47. Sensing the energy track of the base centre with the left palm, patient on the chair.

You will sense that one hand is scanning the centre while the other channels the healing. In this way you are always in a position to compare the energy of two centres. Let your hands be guided to decide how long they need to remain at each centre. You should notice a change in sensation, which coincides with the movement from one centre to the next. As you move from centre to centre, be aware that you are also scanning and working with the central channel, linked to each centre, in the same way. Make a note of your sensations and impressions later to build up your database.

Move both palms to the heart centre, with the right opposite the back.

Move both palms to the solar plexus centre, with the right opposite the back.

Move both palms to the sacral centre, with the right opposite the small of the back.

Move both palms to the base centre, remembering the 45 degree angle of sensation between the two palms (as in Action Point 26).

Move both palms away from the base centre, along the energy track within the aura. Hold the left hand opposite the energy track of the base centre. A final sensing will reveal whether the central channel is balanced or calling for more energy.

All your movements should be slow, gentle and purposeful.

Scanning the five energy centre links

Now move to work with the five energy centre links (see Chapter 8, Seven Sacred Steps). When working with a patient on the chair, select those hand positions that enable you to work comfortably. You may prefer to keep one hand opposite the patient's back, as in the previous scans. You can work at the back or along the front of the patient.

Hold the right palm opposite the base with the left palm opposite the heart. Sense the energetic activity bringing the link to a state of balance.

Move the right palm to the sacral and the left to the throat. Proceed as before.

Move the right palm to the solar plexus and the left to the brow. Proceed as before.

Move the right palm to the heart and the left to the crown. Proceed as before.

Move the right palm to the base and keep the left at the crown. Proceed as before.

Now return to the feet to check the balance of the polarities (as in Action Point 18). This may also be sensed by holding the hands just above each shoulder, if preferred. Observe the patient while you are getting a sense of balance in the patient's field.

The skeletal energy circuit scan

Having completed the scanning and healing of the centres, at an etheric level, proceed with scanning and healing the energy circuits associated with the skeleton.

221

Hold the hands near the top of the head (about 5 to 10cm from the body). Move one hand slowly over the top and down the back of the head to locate where the spine joins the base of the skull. Move your leading (right) hand slowly down the spine until you reach its base in the coccyx, keeping your left at the base of the skull. Sense the energy between your two palms. Slowly bring your left hand down the spine to meet the right at the base.

Remember, the procedure in the skeletal circuit scan is in three parts: your leading hand is scanning and clearing the energy between two 'points'; your two palms hold and sense the balance between the two points; your following hand brings in the new healing energy. Be aware of any resistance to the movement of your hands. In this case, pause and wait for the energy to move your hands.

Remove your hands from the base of the spine to work back at the head and to move down one side of the body (moving with the polarity). If it is the right side, then this is your leading hand. Starting at the head, move slowly down the right side of the face, over the cheek-bones and jaw, to the base of the neck. Follow with the left hand. Move your right hand slowly to the right shoulder and follow with the left. Move your right hand to the elbow and follow with the left. Move your right hand to the wrist and follow with the left. Move your right hand carefully over the fingers and follow with the left. Move your right hand gently out into the aura and follow with the left.

Return to the right shoulder and move your right hand down over the ribs to the right hip. Follow with the left.

Positioned behind the body, move both hands to the base of the spine and move the right hand across to the patient's right hip. Follow with the left. Move the right hand to the right knee and follow with the left. Move the right hand to the ankle and follow with the left. Move the right hand out across the foot and toes. Follow with the left. Move your right hand out into the aura and follow with the left.

Repeat the procedure down the left side of the patient's body, starting at the left side of the head and finishing in the aura by the left foot, as before.

Check the balance of the skeletal energy circuits by holding the palms just above the feet or just above the shoulders, as before. Observe the patient while you are getting a sense of balance and experiencing the condition of the skeleton.

Working at a deeper level

In the first part of the healing procedure, the energy scans have allowed the patient's system to open up and present you with an energetic diagnosis. In the second part, the healing now moves to a deeper level as you intuitively work with this energetic diagnosis. You are effectively asking your hands: 'Where do you need to go now?'

Go back to where you feel you need to, based on the information that your hands have given you. This could be either to an energy centre, the skeletal circuit or somewhere on the physical. Work in that order, treating the centres first.

In the case of a centre, move to where in the field your hands need to go – is it still at an etheric level or has it moved to the emotional or mental? (Recall Action Point 26 when you sensed the location of an energy centre and its activity level). In each case, wait for a change of sensation in your palms, which signals that healing has been given.

After completing this phase of the work, see if your intuition is still directing you somewhere. It might be to the feet, to do some more balancing, or to the crown centre. Here, one hand is held near the crown and the other is held out in the aura. If you feel intuitively that you need to go back to do some more healing, realize that this is a sign of your sensitivity to your patient's needs and soul direction. Each time you 'go back', the healing moves to a deeper level and to a different energetic mode. After each phase, return to the feet to check the balance of the patient.

Closing the healing procedure

The healing procedure ends when you find yourself at the patient's feet for the final time. Stand in front of your patient and hold your hands out to direct to the aura. This is a good point at which to mentally give your thanks.

Give your patient the agreed signal that the healing is over. Gently talk them back to a normal waking state with your hands on their shoulders (or the ankles/feet), just as they were when you talked them into the relaxation state at the beginning. Once they seem to be coming back, move to where they can see you. Encourage them to open their eyes, when they feel ready, and to spend a moment taking in where they are. Many patients feel the need to hold your hand at this point. Be ready for this, as it is an important signal that you are there for them and that they have returned safely to their body.

When you are sure they are back (in their body), check that their eyes are taking in their surroundings and assist them to the meeting chair where the session began.

Concluding the session

Some patients are very thirsty and need a drink. Encourage them to sip the water slowly.

Ask them if there is anything they would like to say or if they have any questions. Of course it is quite all right if they do not have anything to say. Some patients like to ask about what they experienced – offer them the space to do this. Remember that this second talking period is still part of the session and helps to ground the patient's experience in the here and now.

Discuss any homework and make the next appointment, if this is appropriate. Assure the patient that the effects of the healing will continue even when they have left the therapy room.

The whole session has taken about an hour. The talking element at the beginning and the end may well take half an hour altogether.

After the patient has left, clear the chair(s) and the couch as well as yourself. This can be done by visualizing light clearing the furniture, your energy field and the energy of the room.

Clearing returns yourself and the space to the same energetic condition as when you started. This is important if you are going to work with another patient. The Sacred Meeting has been completed. How do you feel?

THE THOROUGHNESS OF THE SOUL-BASED APPROACH

We tell Sally's story to illustrate the thoroughness of the soul-based approach. Here, the healer needed to be open to soul-guidance in order to work effectively with the energetic diagnosis revealed in the first part of the healing procedure.

Six months after surgery for a hysterectomy, Sally was experiencing lower abdominal pain. The pain would often travel down her right leg, making sitting and walking uncomfortable. Further medical investigation proved inconclusive. She was told to get on with her life.

With work becoming virtually impossible because of the pain, Sally thought she would try healing, for her father had been interested in healing before his death three years previously.

The scans revealed a damaged energy circuit from the base of the spine to the right hip. This was cutting off energy to the right leg. The base, sacral, heart and throat centres were all calling for energy and were exhibiting varying degrees of malfunction. Over the next four weeks the pain began to ease as the functioning of the centres was restored and the energy circuits repaired.

In the following session, Sally seemed more deeply relaxed – she was accessing her healing dream. During her sleep Sally's hands rose to her throat and then gently returned to her sides. She remained in a deep sleep and showed no sign of being aware of the movement of her hands. When Sally awoke she reached up to her throat saying, 'I saw my father. We were in a jewellery shop and he bought me a beautiful necklace. I could see it so clearly. It had rubies, emeralds, sapphires and an orange stone I don't know the name of. Dad helped me put it on straight away. I could feel it.' She pointed to her throat, 'I was wearing it right here. It might sound crazy but I feel as if it's still here even though I can't see it.'

'This feels very different,' she said pointing to her lower abdomen. 'The pain is completely gone. I've been healed. My father has healed me!' she said excitedly.

From that session Sally was indeed free from pain. Her father had found a way of practising healing after all. His gift of the jewelled necklace completely matched the centres needing healing.

Hearing Sally's story, you would gather that surgery had affected the related energy centre (the sacral) as well as the energy circuit of the lower skeleton. Note how the damaged sacral was impacting on the lower abdomen.

The base centre was found to be involved with the problem in the pelvis and right leg, and further investigation revealed that the sacral link centre, the throat, also needed healing. Interestingly, her father in spirit worked particularly with the throat centre by giving her a necklace. The colours of the necklace jewels also corroborated the energetic diagnosis that the base-heart (red/green) and sacral-throat (orange/blue) links had been affected.

Sally's story also demonstrates a function of the healing sleep. She not only meets up with her father, but has confirmation of the continuity of life and of his love for her when he is directly involved in her healing. Thus, as well as the intuitive work on the energy centres and circuits, Sally needed this experience to complete her healing.

The Place Of Love, Peace And Light In The Session

Before finishing this chapter, let's pause a moment to see where Love, Peace and Light have fitted into the Sacred Meeting.

The Love is the respect for the patient, shown by the soul-centred and unconditional positive regard for the patient by the healer. Love is also present in the effort the healer has made to create the sacred space for the work. Peace enters through the atmosphere created by the healer and the breathing and relaxation exercises or procedures which allow the patient to feel safe, cared for and enveloped by the Love. There is outer peace in the room and inner peace in the healer and the patient. The patient begins to adjust to the energetic atmosphere of the sacred space. Once there is this Love and Peace, Light, in the form of healing, will follow.

We have included a number of patient stories throughout the book, to show you the range of possibilities for helping others, which the soul-based approach provides. We hope that they will inspire you to work this way or to integrate the soul-based approach into your own practice.

You will need to find time to make notes about your sessions, your findings and experiences, and any homework that you have given your patient. In the next chapter we make some suggestions on how you can go about this.

Beyond The Healing Session

15

Working Outside the Healing Session

The healing effect does indeed carry on after a session is over and this will reinforce a sense of continuity in the patient between sessions. There are various things you or the patient will need to do, which may well form part of this pattern of continuity. The back-up work you do outside the session ensures your professional approach to practice and also your soul-based approach, which encourages respect for yourself as well as your patient.

THE HEALER

Writing up the session

We do not recommend that you make a tape recording during the session for later reference. Even if your patient agrees to this, you will both be conscious of it and this will interfere with the authentic nature of the meeting.

But it is important for any practitioner to make notes about the therapy sessions, bearing in mind that, by law, these notes may be accessed by the patient on request. Patient confidentiality is paramount. Stored patient details are subject to the Data Protection Act, the contents of which you should be aware.

We advise against note-taking during the session. This can act as a block to communication and prevents you from being fully present with your patient as your focus shifts to note-taking. Post-session notes should be brief and to the point, stating what actually took place. Include what procedures were used, breathing, relaxation and any other instructions, any music used, their effects and any patient homework suggested. Be sparing with your opinions and any subjective descriptions.

If you are going to see a patient for more than a few sessions you should vary your instructions, and those techniques that are additional to the healing procedure, so that there is variety and something new for the patient. So why not think about your 'repertoire'?

If you refer the patient to another practitioner, for whatever reason, this should be in your session notes (see below).

Evaluating the session

Since this is a subjective exercise, it may not have a place in your session notes, but you should still spend some time evaluating the energetic process of the session and its effects on the patient. Recall the state of the patient on arrival and at departure. Did the scans and your healing procedures corroborate the patient's story? Did your interventions help to facilitate the patient to tell their story? Note where this occurred and where it may not have.

In your evaluation, you make an honest assessment of whether your patient needs other kinds of help you cannot offer. Make sure you are in a position to refer patients on if this is the case. You need to have a list of other practitioners and health care professionals to whom you can refer or seek guidance from. In this way you contribute to creating the healing community.

Know your limitations. Do you need to acquire some new skills or new knowledge – for example, counselling skills? Allow your intuition to guide you about this.

Finally, is there anything you could have done differently?

Your energetic diagnosis

Through your work with the scans, and other intuitive information gained during the talking elements of the session, you are able to make an energetic diagnosis about your patient. This means that you have knowledge about the current state of the person in terms of their subtle energy system. This is not a medical diagnosis and should not be used as a talking point with patients, nor should it ever influence how you view them.

Energetic diagnosis should never be identified as a statement about a person. Rather it is a statement of your awareness, perceptions and impressions during the healing session at that point in time.

Pondering the session

After the session, take time to ponder: What has this soul (what have these souls) been saying to me today? Because of Oneness, you are learning from your patient. You are part of their process and they are part of yours. In pondering the sessions, you are using mind, memory and your feelings, as well as intuition, to contemplate messages from soul.

It is good to review your sessions at the end of a week or month. You might ask yourself: Why are these people finding their way to me? What messages are they offering me? What is my attention being drawn to?

Creating a database

Every healing session is a gift from your patient, enabling you to gain experience and knowledge, to increase your awareness and to become a hollow bone. During the session, and often in between sessions, your brow centre supplies you with a vast amount of perceptual data that you should log in some way. This helps you to build your own database about what certain perceptions, sensations and impressions mean to *you*.

Throughout this book, we have encouraged you to create your own database about your energetic experiences and in any situation where you are developing awareness. This is important because no two healers experience the same perceptions in the same situation (because we are humans at different stages of awareness and development, not robots).

For this reason you should be wary of comparing yourself with others and of taking the word of any author or teacher without checking what they say for yourself. Remember the lesson of the throat centre – be authentic. Get used to trusting your inner judgement, knowing that if you are heart-centred all will be well.

It can be useful to be sceptical if this encourages you to be scientific – to gather data and to compare it with the 'facts' of the case, the patient's story and progress.

Referring on and useful information

Keep lists of a range of complementary therapists working in your area, with addresses and telephone numbers. Ideally the patient should be able to take such a list with them.

Details of support groups functioning in your locality with the name and telephone number of the organiser can help the patient feel less isolated. Such groups allow patients to talk with others about what it is they are experiencing. Patients report feeling great benefit from spending time with others who understand what may be happening and who are not members of their family! Such support groups provide a vital element of the healing community.

Patients may benefit from joining classes in meditation, relaxation, t'ai chi, yoga, etc., which may be offered as part of their local authority adult education scheme or run privately.

Communication is a two-way process. Patients are a mine of information. Stay alert during conversations for details of activities in your area, which may serve as additions to your lists.

We all respond to books that are inspiring, uplifting or shed light on experience. Have lists of available texts, organized under topics such as healing, spirituality, complementary medicine, women's health, women's studies, shamanism and biographies of inspiring people.

Patients may ask for information about the music played in the healing sessions. Have ready the details so that they may obtain a copy. Some patients report that they relive the healing session just by playing the music. The music played may be a soothing antidote to much of the noise the patient is otherwise exposed to.

Healer support groups

The healer is part of the community. It is important, therefore, not to become isolated and to find support for your work. The healer support group is designed to do this and it can be structured in any way that suits group members. It could take the form of simple networking, for example.

Such groups have an energy that is nourishing, helping to build friendships, a joint sense of purpose, a discussion base about work situations and creating space for peer supervision. If there is no group near you, why not start one yourself?

When the group allows itself to be soul-guided, it will evolve in ways that help every member of the group and the group as a whole. Here is an ideal place for simple ceremony, celebration and enjoyment of this aspect of the healing life.

Your journal

Keep your journal going and make sure it is lively and fun. This is your private place where you can do and say what you like. Subjects you might consider are: What is happening in your life and in the life of the world that seems significant to you? How are life events matching your awareness work, your centring and healing practice? How are you feeling and how do you interact with other spiritual healers or therapists? Are there plenty of friends who have nothing to do with the world of healing?

THE PATIENT

Building on the session

Often patients ask if there is anything they can do to build on what we are doing in the healing session. The answer is always, yes, a great deal.

Whatever exercise has been introduced in the session can safely be continued at home. Responding to the patient's request for 'homework' harnesses their interest in self-healing and begins the process of building a range of self-help techniques, which continue to support good practice long after the period of healing has finished.

Breathing and relaxation

Most patients will benefit from continuing the basic breathing and relaxation exercises introduced. In today's busy lifestyle breathing and relaxation go a long way towards protecting against the harmful effects of stress. Many people do not breathe properly and many do not know how to relax.

Breathing exercises can include full breath breathing, rhythmic breathing or a combination of both.

Relaxation exercises can include full body relaxation and mental relaxation. (All these breathing and relaxation exercises can be found in Chapter 11, Sacred Tools: Breathing and Relaxation).

Working with colour

Patients can be introduced to the vibratory colours of the subtle energy centres and then encouraged to practise breathing the relevant colour into the centre and body part influenced by that centre. The colour is then breathed out into the aura. The healer suggests which centres are related to the condition. Here are some examples:

- The sacral centre (orange) is related to lower back trouble.
- One woman bought a turquoise necklace and earrings for the condition affecting her throat and ears (throat centre).
- One of the colours most of us need is green, the great balancer. This is why it is good to go out into nature to be with this colour. The combination of sun, blue sky and green fields or trees is particularly effective. The balancing is always enhanced when the patient consciously breathes the colour into the system, via the heart centre.

Protecting the energy centres

Much energy is lost through emotional situations. Patients can be encouraged to protect the principal vitality energy centre, the solar plexus, by imagining a large golden disc (at least the size of a large dinner plate) covering the solar plexus area, extending from the top of the navel to just below the breast bone. Placing the hand on the body to position the disc reinforces the intention of protection. A second disc may be added to the back, again sensing where exactly it needs to go. It will sit opposite the front disc.

Patients have reported noticing how the disc loses its brightness after a busy day at the office and needs a polish, which they do mentally. In the early stages of developing respect for the subtle aspects of being, the positioning of

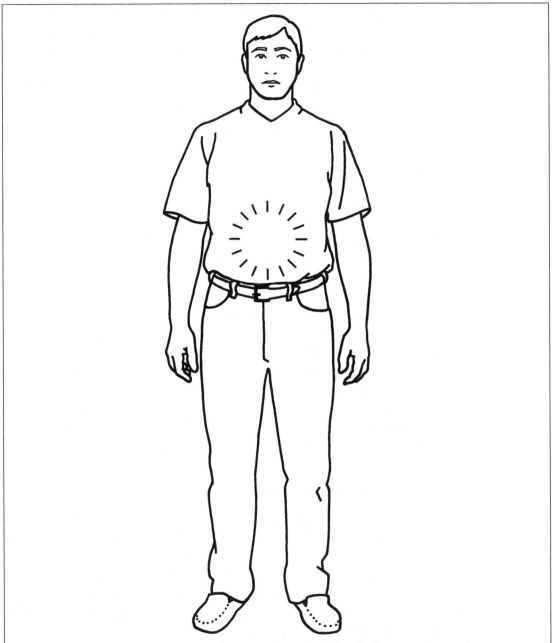

Figure 48. The Solar Disc. Visualizing a disc of golden light covering and protecting the solar plexus centre.

the disc is practised daily. It is an effective exercise to prevent energy drain and loss through this major centre. When patients are readjusting their systems through healing, they need to conserve and protect their energies.

Some patients are able to sense which energy centres become affected by inharmonious situations and adapt the protective disc technique by matching colour to centre.

Protecting the energy field

Aura protection helps the patient be less vulnerable to the effects of disruptive energy in the environment, at work or at home.

Patients are encouraged to clear their energy system at the end of the day. They then begin the next day by placing a sphere of light around themselves, starting at the heels with the in-breath, drawing the light up the back, pausing at the top of the head and with the out-breath projecting the bubble down the front of the body, reaching under the toes and feet. This may be repeated from the left to the right of the body. Some patients need this second sweep of energy protection to feel 'enclosed' within the sphere of light. Patients often report seeing the light sphere as a colour. This always relates to what they are needing at the time, and can be an empowering and exciting discovery for the individual (see Action Points 8 and 9).

When patients talk about having to face a difficult scenario, they are encouraged to use the protective sphere technique described above. These protective measures may be implemented in seconds in response to any signal that disruptive energies are present.

Working creatively with healing session experiences

During the healing sleep patients often intuitively see or know something of relevance to their current state and/or healing.

Patients may revisit past experiences, replay current scenarios or access obscure images and symbols. Whatever the experience, patients are able to describe it vividly. To reinforce this profound means of accessing one's own healing power, patients are encouraged to illustrate their experience in some way. This may be a drawing, a painting, a collage, something three-dimensional, etc. No artistic expertise is required. Some patients have produced beautiful illustrations that serve as mandalas for their meditation practice. In the act of illustrating the experience, additional information is often released to the patient. Patients are encouraged to bring their art work to the next session and to discuss it if they wish. Some patients ask for their art work to be placed alongside them on the healing couch.

The invitation to illustrate experience is often met with the response, 'Oh, I couldn't do that, I'm no artist. I haven't done anything like that since I was at school'. But at the same time a glint in the eye says that an aspect of them relishes the permission to be creative! A major healing exercise is being undertaken with significant release of stored material, especially via the sacral and throat chakras. There will be visual clues in the work created about the activity of other chakras.

Taking care

'Look after yourself' are often the last words a patient will hear as they leave the healing session.

However, when the patient is cut off from their feelings of self-worth or self-care, this phrase may have little or no meaning for them and is met with a blank look. For some the phrase comes as a total surprise. For others the response is 'Yes, I know', as if they have been reminded of something they had forgotten or not considered to be part of their responsibility to themselves as a demonstration of the love they have for themselves.

There are many patients who undermine the effectiveness of the healing session by not looking after themselves. Lifestyle, poor diet and lack of exercise will need to be addressed. For this reason it is necessary to have details of professionals to hand to which reference and referrals can be made.

For many people who cannot get to a healer, a request for distant healing is a way of looking after themselves. Though it may always be a useful adjunct to the healing sessions, distant healing is a complete way of working, in its own right, which we describe in the next chapter.

16

Distant Healing

We always tell groups of trainee healers how distant healing – healing with the person at a distance, as opposed to contact healing when the patient is there – is an excellent way to begin to practise as a healer. You do not need to have a healing practice, be near a healing centre or find yourself some patients. You will soon get a feel for the work and start to understand what part your hands want to play in it. It is a very good way of getting to know your own healing signals and beginning to build your database about this.

While you work as a distant healer, you will learn a lot about healing and your work is just as valid as any contact work.

You do not need to go looking for patients. The law of attraction means that people will seek your help because the time is right for both of you to meet, as your individual paths cross. This is the moment of the Sacred Meeting and it has been arranged at a soul level with the agreement of all concerned. But distant healing, too, when carried out with the soul-based approach, is another form of Sacred Meeting and is a moment of holy synchronicity.

Working Unconditionally

In its simplest form, distant healing can be a prayer asking that healing will be sent to the person who needs it. The request should be made unconditionally so that healing is directed to where it is needed and not where we, with limited knowledge and understanding, think it should be directed. In other words, we ask for healing for the person without limiting our request to something like 'Please cure her cancer'.

However, as we have emphasized in this book, Spiritual Healing encourages us to realize that we are soul, that we are Oneness. So *who* or *what* are we praying to? Through the soul-based approach, we are able to take responsibility for doing the work ourselves. This honours the fact that the person is the soul and not the body, and that it is the soul that directs the healing energies. It also honours the soul's deeper reasons for the condition, which we, on a personality level, know nothing about.

If a person asks for distant healing for themselves, or for another, for a specific condition, allow them to descibe it to you and to talk about it in the way *they* need to. This is part of the healing process and will not prevent you from working unconditionally.

The Distant Healing Circle

We hope there will come a time when distant healing groups are set up all over the world, in every town and in every country. Group energy is particularly effective in creating the conditions for distant healing. The distant healing circle is an opportunity to meet on a regular basis, as a group of healers or like-minded people, to do service for the community and the wider world.

The next Action Point is a simple way of meeting as a group to send distant healing. If you are working by yourself or with a partner, the procedure can be adapted accordingly.

You will need a group leader/facilitator each time and every member of the group should take a turn at this. It is helpful to bring either a list of requests for healing or a list of those who have intuitively come to mind. The length of your list will be dictated by the time you have together. A list of about ten names should suffice.

It is especially important in this new century to always include healing for peace, healing for planet Earth and the Earth family.

ACTION POINT 49 The Distant Healing Circle

Developmental tool – learning to work with the energies of Spiritual Healing at a distance from the patient, within the context of a group.

Have a circle of chairs in the centre of which is a small table with a candle and some matches. Members might like to add personal items symbolizing healing. Disconnect all telephones. Make sure everyone has their list of people, animals, situations, etc. The group leader should help the group to attune and then facilitate the distant healing.

- The group sits in a circle with feet flat on the floor and their hands, palms up, on their thighs or in their laps without linking. Use the breath to calm and relax the body.

- Let go of any worries or anxieties (which may be uppermost in your mind since compiling your distant healing list) with the out-breath, through the open mouth. Close your mouth when you feel centred and breathe normally. Check that the body is relaxed, including the back of the neck, the shoulders and pelvis. Close your eyes and allow the calm silence to settle upon the group.

- Light the candle and dedicate the light to the work of the distant healing circle. Ask for protection and the guidance of soul.

- See the light of the candle as the light of the soul and breathe it into the heart centre.

- Now pass the energy in your heart centre to the person on your left until you are all linked together. Intuitively, you may have to wait to gather your heart energy before you can pass it on. The group leader should be aware of this and allow enough time for group linking, for this is the foundation of the healing circle.

- The leader expresses the purpose of the meeting and gives thanks for the opportunity to be of service.

- Aware of the light in the heart centre, see this light extending from you to the centre of the circle. As every member extends their light it becomes the light of healing.

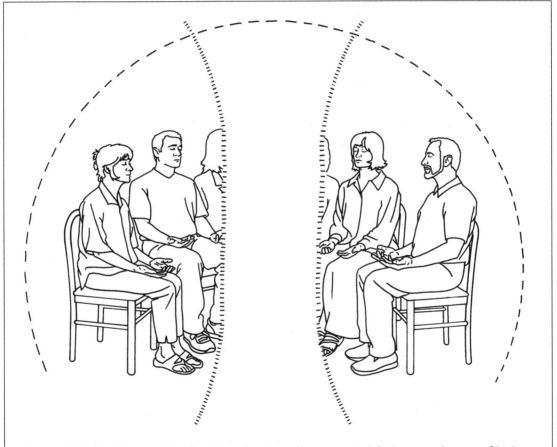

Figure 49. The Distant Healing Circle. Members are visualizing a column of light in the centre.

- The leader reads out their list, asking for healing for each person named, knowing that they will be put or held in the light. A simple form of this could be, 'I ask for healing for (name) ...'. The leader indicates that they have completed their list with a signal such as 'thank you'.

- The person on their left then reads out their list and repeats the conclusion signal. Follow this procedure until everyone has read out their list. The leader should then indicate to the circle that, if other names have come to anyone's mind, now is the time to mention them.

- By watching your inner screen (above the brow), you may 'see' these people or you may not. It is important to know that your intention, motivated by love, has put them in the light of healing.

- As you sit together in the silence, retain your awareness of the light in the centre. See if your inner screen shows you what is happening to the light.

- The leader may now close the circle. As you blow out the candle, you can send the light out to where it is needed – a strife-ridden place, an environment under threat, and so on.

- Discuss the work of the circle as a group. Share experiences and queries to consolidate your learning.

- This exercise could be followed by a group meditation. If not, carry out the closing down and protection exercises given in Chapter 5, A Way of Being, before you disperse.

EMPOWERMENT AND RESPONSIBILITY

When people ask for your help as a distant healer, ask them in return to let you know how they, or the requested person, are getting on after a period of two to four weeks. Feedback is essential so that you can monitor what happens. It also encourages people to take responsibility for their requests.

The patient can be further empowered by joining in. Ideally, this should be at the same time as the healing is being sent, but it is not crucial, as we shall explain shortly. Ask them to sit or lie quietly at the time you will be sending out to them. Ask them to relax and visualize a sphere of protecting light around them. They should remain like this for 15 minutes.

Keep a record of all distant healing requests and any feedback that you receive.

Some healers work entirely in this way and find it as effective in many cases as contact healing. All cases will benefit from distant healing, but bear in mind that some people need the talking element of the healing session in order for deep healing to take place.

SITUATIONS WHEN DISTANT HEALING IS CALLED FOR

Distant healing is the best way of working when people cannot travel, when they are confined for various reasons, when they are suffering from a contagious disease, or a mental or behavioural condition that prevents contact. If the person cannot get to you or you to them, you can always offer distant healing.

Sometimes a person would never go for healing, but a friend or relative wants to help them. It will not be intrusive if the distant healer is working the soul-based way and asks for healing for that person without specifying any condition. It will then be up to the recipient, at a soul level, to decide how they will use the energies. If the person does not make use of them, the energies will flow on to where they can be used.

Because energy follows thought, it travels at the level of that thought. So it can be very intrusive to send something conditional to another person when they have not asked for your help. For example, a friend tells you that they have heard of an aquaintance who has been diagnosed HIV positive. 'We should not only send some healing in case he develops AIDS, he probably needs help for his lifestyle as well,' says your friend. When an initial impulse of love becomes distorted by mind-based judgement, this energy, travelling at the level of such thoughts, may be unwanted, unnecessary, or ineffective.

This is why the healer does not attempt to direct healing energy to any aspect or level of a person (even though it is possible to do so), neither can their work involve any sort of judgement.

How Distant Healing Works

Healing energies come from the Source of all energy. This means that they originate outside the space/time frame of the physical and so are not governed by its laws until they enter this level. Thus, they can travel to where they are needed, at any distance, in an instant. Once the soul becomes aware of the energies moving into its field, it directs them to the appropriate level.

Sometimes the energy will reach the physical instantly and bring about change. Sometimes energy will be needed on a subtle level first and change may be seen here. Just as in contact healing, where healing energies are directed depends on a number of factors, such as the cause of the condition, the soul's journey or the state of readiness for change in the person.

Health is not an isolated condition of the body, but a function of the harmony of our total being of body, emotion, mind and spirit. So there can be no 'right' or 'wrong', 'good' or 'bad' condition. Soul always honours the body consciousness and seeks to co-operate with it, rather than to manipulate it.

The Astral Level And Healing

It is also common for healers to work on the astral level. The word *astral* is derived from the Latin and Greek for 'star' (*astron*). We sleep when the stars are out, hence 'astral travelling' has come to mean travelling during the sleep state, in your 'astral body', on the 'astral level'. The so-called astral level is any level of being outside of the physical when you are in your astral body – which can happen at any time.

When you consider that we all leave our bodies during sleep, the fact of astral travelling is understandable and not so surprising. But it means that patients frequently report healers appearing in their dreams and in their waking state, talking to them and giving them healing of various kinds. Naturally, this is not just something healers do, we all do it, but most of us just do not seem to retain the conscious memory of it.

Soul is able to travel like this, outside the physical level, through its creation, the astral body. This vehicle has a frequency band which at its lowest range lies between the etheric and the emotional energy zones. In a similar fashion to when we are in the physical body, we have a containment

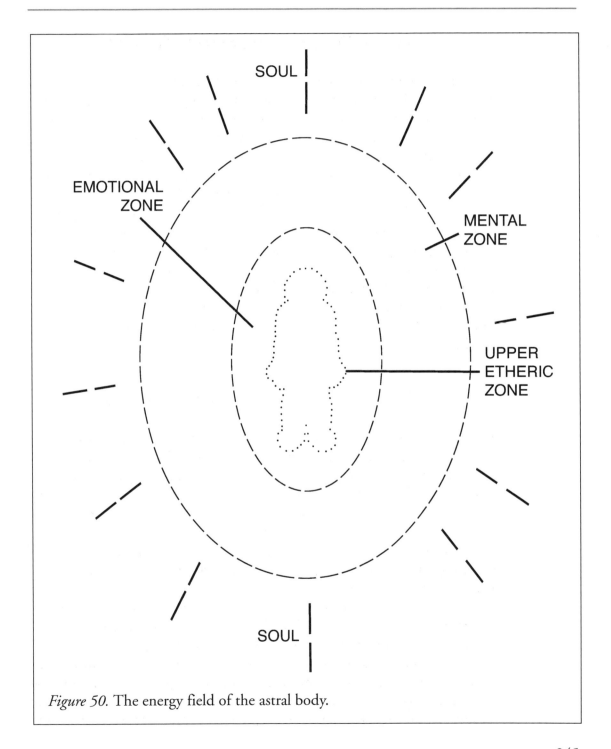

Figure 50. The energy field of the astral body.

vehicle (the astral) with energetic links to the etheric, and the energy zones of the emotional, mental and soul. A diagram of the aura of the astral body would show that the physical and 'lower' etheric levels are not present.

Some healers are able to move on to the astral level to carry out distant healing during their waking state. This may be a conscious or unconscious experience. So a person may describe how the healer appeared to them, yet the healer has no waking knowledge of this.

Conscious astral level healing can occur in two basic ways when the healer sits for distant healing. They find that they can either 'travel' (in their astral body) to the person needing help or that person is brought to them in their astral body. Some distant healers like to work this way, especially when there is an emergency call for help. It is possibe to train yourself to travel in your astral body, but most healers have not reached this state of conscious control over their astral movements and are happy to rely on soul-guidance as to how or when the travelling will take place.

Maybe you are happy to go with the flow of soul too. To find out, the next Action Point is designed to help you to begin conscious astral level healing.

ACTION POINT 50 Astral Level Healing

Developmental tool – preparing to work with the energies of Sacred Healing on the astral level of existence.

Recommended for group experience only until confident and proficient to work this way alone.

- Prepare yourself on all levels for distant healing, as in Action Point 49. Ask to be guided by soul, accepting what soul directs (whether or not you will be doing any healing at the astral level).

- Take the first request on your distant healing list and ask to be used as a channel for healing for this person. Mention them by name because the vibration of the name strengthens the link (of the Healing Triangle – see Figure 8 in Chapter 6, Preparing Sacred Space).

- Close your eyes, relax and wait quietly and patiently to see if you become aware that the person is there in front of you.

- If you have been 'taken' to the person, or they have been brought to you, you will sense them in front of you. This becomes easier when you are able to relax, accept soul-guidance and accept that it is possible for this to happen. You will also be able to sense whether the person, child, baby, or animal is lying or sitting in front of you and how the body is oriented. Mentally make sure that you are comfortably oriented with them to carry out what needs to be done. As in contact healing, use your intuition, your soul-guidance that is directing you, to sense where your hands want to go.

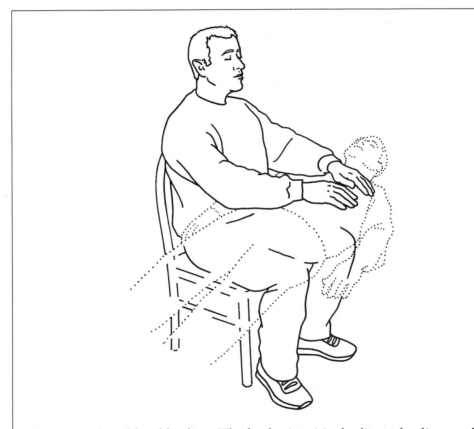

Figure 51. Astral level healing. The healer intuitively directs healing to the person as if he is physically present.

- Let's take an example as explanation. Your help has been requested for a young man who has had an operation on his chest. In this case, once you are aware of his astral body in front of you, you will feel drawn to put your hands over the area in question. If this is what he needs, you will feel healing energy leave your hands — or whatever sign that tells you that you are working. Keep them there until you feel a change in the flow that tells you the healing is complete. Wait for your guidance to see if you need to give healing elsewhere. There may be a centre involved, for example, or you may need to go somewhere other than the chest.

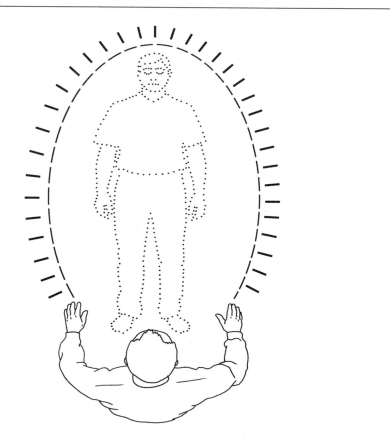

Figure 52. Astral level healing. The sphere of protection. The healer intuitively directs a sphere of light to surround the distant healing patient before closing the session.

- The energetic happenings in your hands are confirmation that this is not taking place in your imagination. A person with developed perceptions would be able to sense or 'see' what was going on and confirm that you were working this way. You are in a sacred space doing sacred work.

- When you have completed your work with that person, thank them at a soul level and surround them with a protective sphere of light. This may be done mentally or by moving your hands gently to make a sphere around the body.

- The distant healing patient then returns to their physical body or the healer does the same. The healer may remain in the astral body state to receive the next patient in this way. In some cases you both return to your physical bodies.

- Break the link with the patient by visualizing clearing light washing over your upraised palms. You can now proceed to the next person on the list.

If, during an astral level healing, you feel you are no longer sitting in your chair but standing over or by the patient, this signals that you have travelled to them. Keep relaxed and proceed as described. You are quite safe and can move out of this state whenever you like.

We recommend that you start to work this way with one patient at a time and build up to six at any one session, unless guided otherwise. You need to feel totally comfortable and build up your confidence so that you do not get tired by the level of focused effort needed to work this way.

Keep a note of your impressions and make sure you get some feedback about your work. If you intend to work as an astral healer on a regular basis, keep a record of what happens, just as you would with a contact patient.

Ways Of Working Together

It is good to compare notes with another healer or healers who are working this way. Networking allows you to share and gain knowledge and insight from the experience of others. It acts as a form of peer supervision and helps to keep everyone's 'feet on the ground'.

A way of networking and including peer supervision is to work on the astral level with a group or healing circle. You will need a group leader/facilitator each time and every member of the group should take a turn at this. The group should have one list you have compiled together. The length of your list will be dictated by the time you have together, but should be no more than six to ten tasks, unless you are intuitively guided otherwise. It is important to always include some work on a planetary situation or for the Earth family. Read through the exercise carefully, noting that you need to elect a leader and a set of 'nominees' for each meeting (see below).

ACTION POINT 51 Astral Level Healing Circle

Developmental tool – exploring working with the energies of Spiritual Healing on the astral level, within the energetic structure of group consciousness.

Have a circle of chairs, in the centre of which is a candle that can be safely placed on the floor. Disconnect all telephones. The group leader should help the group to attune and then facilitate the distant healing by announcing who or what is on the list of tasks.

- The group sits in a circle with feet flat on the floor and their hands, palms up, on their thighs or in their laps without linking. Use the breath to calm and relax the body. Let go of any worries or anxieties (which may be uppermost in your mind since compiling your distant healing list) with the out-breath, through the open mouth. Close your mouth when you feel centred and breathe normally. Check that the body is relaxed, including the back of the neck, the shoulders and pelvis. Close your eyes and allow the calm silence to settle upon the group.

- Light the candle and dedicate the light to the work of the distant healing circle. Ask for protection and the guidance of soul.

- See the light of the candle as the light of the soul and breathe it into the heart centre.

- Now pass the energy in your heart centre to the person on your left, until you are all linked together. Intuitively, you may have to wait to gather your heart energy before you can pass it on. The group leader should be aware of this and allow enough time for group linking, for this is the foundation of the healing circle.

- The leader expresses the purpose of the meeting and gives thanks for the opportunity to be of service.

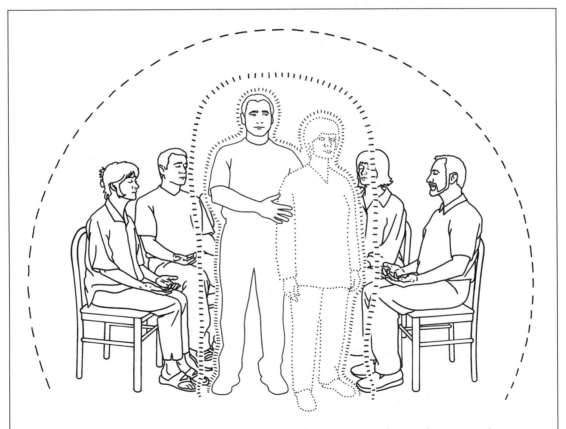

Figure 53. The Astral Level Healing Circle. The nominated member is working on a patient who is present in their astral body.

- Be aware of the light in the heart centre; see this light extending from you to the centre of the circle. As every member extends their light it becomes the light of healing.

- The leader annouces the first task by praying: 'We ask to be used as channels of healing for ... (name of the first person/animal/situation, etc. on the list, which we will term 'the patient').

- The group waits for the patient to appear (to their inner vision) in the centre of the circle. As soon as the nominated member is aware of this, the nominee works on the patient, as in Action Point 50. The rest of the group contribute to the healing by sitting in awareness with upraised palms. Energy will be beamed from their palms to the patient in the centre.

- Other group members may feel intuitively that they need to use their hands also. This should only occur once the nominated member has begun to work.

- The leader should monitor group activity. Work is completed on the first named person when the nominated member has ceased hand activity and returned them to the resting position. The leader should indicate this to the group with a gentle signal, such as a bell or with the words, 'We have completed the work for (name) ...'. The group should all return their hands to the resting position.

- The leader then announces the next task and the group proceeds as before, with a different nominee each time.

- When the list is complete, the leader should indicate this to the group. Sit together in the silence for a few moments before closing the circle.

- Send the light out. You may want to link hands or exchange hugs as a way of celebrating your heart-based work together.

- Discuss the work as a group. Share experiences and queries to consolidate your learning.

The astral level healing circle could be followed by a group meditation. If not, carry out the closing down and protection exercises described in Chapter 5, A Way of Being, before you disperse.

A common request for distant healing is to help the terminally ill to pass over or to help the bereaved who are left behind. Families also ask for help when a baby is expected and the healing will be directed to the mother, the incoming soul and to the nursing team involved. In this sense, distant healing very often plays a part in the sacred rituals of birth and death – rituals each of us will celebrate at some time.

The
Celebrations

17

Sacred Rituals

Our birth is but a sleep and a forgetting:
The Soul that rises with us, our life's star,
Hath had elsewhere its setting,
And cometh from afar:
Not in entire forgetfulness,
And not in utter nakedness,
But trailing clouds of glory do we come
From God, who is our home

William Wordsworth,
Intimations of immortality from recollections of early childhood (1803)

The pattern of our first and last breaths marks the beginning and end of each soul's life journey. They are the simple, but profound rituals that celebrate our life on Earth.

When the incoming being takes in the life force with the first intake of breath, they signal to their ancestors that they have come to breathe the same breath as them and to be a part of Earth life for a while. At the end of the journey, the person gives out their last breath to those they leave behind and to those who are to come.

We celebrate birth, but choose to forget that death is our way back to the light. For a very long time, the rituals of the incoming and outgoing breath have placed Earth life at the centre of human experience. It is now time for the world to place soul at the centre of life, so that death too can be a celebratory ritual.

We tell Julia's story because, when she was very ill, she wanted to place soul at the centre of her life. It has so much to say that is life-enhancing about the event most people dread. So this is our way of thanking her.

I first spoke to Julia on a Sunday. It had been a day of celebration, joining with the local community at the naming ceremony of recently arrived twins. Later that evening the phone rang. A softly spoken woman said, 'I'm looking for someone to help me die. Can you teach me about dying? I've had cancer for seven years and I've been in remission twice but it all feels different this time. I feel different. My consultant has told me there's nothing more to be done. I have six months to live. But I don't want to die like my mother – she was terrified and struggled to hold on to life ...' . She paused.

'I'm here,' I said.

'Something tells me it doesn't have to be like that. I just feel it can be different but I don't know what to do or how to go about it.'

Two days later, Julia and I explored the issue of death within the context of Spiritual Healing, where death is as much a celebration as birth. We agreed to undertake a journey together in which I would help Julia prepare for her passing from this life into the next. I would accompany her until she signalled that she was ready to continue her journey alone.

We met twice weekly, when Julia would use the healing sessions to practise leaving her physical body. During the deep relaxation state of her healing sleeps she found herself reviewing her life. She was reminded of all the wonderful experiences life had presented. She accessed issues of 'unfinished business' and set about 'clearing the slate' between sessions. This gentle woman was showing herself how to celebrate her life and at the same time to let go of it. Julia's appearance began to change – she looked well and at times glowed after our healing sessions together.

Five months had passed when Julia announced she would like her husband and two teenage children to witness her healing sessions so that they could see her as she would be when she died. 'I think I've got the idea of it now.'

Her husband Brian accompanied her at the next session. Julia slipped effortlessly into her healing sleep and left her physical body lying on the couch. I signalled to Brian that she had gone. 'I know,' he whispered. 'I saw her – she showed me.' On her return Julia and a tearful Brian agreed that the children could attend. Brian said he had the same feeling watching Julia leaving her body as when he had watched the birth of their twins. It was wonderful, but difficult to explain.

Brian continued to accompany Julia for the next month when she felt this phase of her journey was drawing to an end. Now it was important for the children to be present. The next week, two nervous teenagers watched Julia's healing session, holding hands with their father as he whispered reassurances. Mum relaxed, slept and journeyed beyond the physical. On her return she shared her experience of beauty and light with her husband and children. She told them how she could see us all in the room and how she could see her body lying on the couch, yet she 'wasn't there'. She lovingly explained that she would always be there for them but in a different way. The healing for the family had begun.

It was a Sunday night again when a call came from Julia. This time her voice seemed distant. 'I've packed my bags and I'm all ready so I'm organizing my send-off party. Can you come?' she laughed. 'Of course,' I replied. 'I wouldn't miss it for the world.'

Arriving at Julia's house, I was met by Brian and the children. There was a mixture of celebration and sadness in the air. As we hugged each other, Brian whispered, 'This is it.'

Julia was in bed surrounded with flowers and candles. She smiled. 'This is where our journey ends. It's time to take our different paths – thank you.' The family said their goodbyes.

'Goodbye, Julia.' I kissed her forehead and sat with my palms directing healing to her.

Time passed. She stirred only once to say that she could see her mother. Her face was lit by a smile that filled the room. She was on her way. Eventually Julia slipped out of her body as she had done so many times before. But this time there would be no return.

Events in Julia's life brought her to the point where she had to face her own death. She did not want it to be a distressingly futile attempt to cling on to life, but her conscious decision about how it was to happen. She realized that she could learn how to die, and found that it could be done with grace and dignity.

Perhaps Julia's story will show you the wisdom of meditating on your own death, in being ready for death, in realizing that it is part of your journey. Her story tells us that there are essential preparations for all of us, especially if we are going to be in the presence of the dying and if we are going to work with the dying in a healing capacity. We cannot understand our role if we have not addressed the fact of our own death, the possibility of readiness and the place of death in our own soul journey.

So let us begin with a contemplation that will help us to gain some of the understanding we seek.

ACTION POINT 52 Contemplation – Life to Death to Life

Developmental tool – experiencing the sacred rituals of life, death and rebirth; accessing the vital energies contained within the rituals.

This exercise may be used for self-healing, but should be carried out with a partner.

Your partner will need to be sensitive to your progress through the exercise and its impact upon you. Instructions should be given in a soft, calm voice, allowing plenty of time for experiencing. Your partner will hold (maintain) the energetic space for you during your 'journeying'.

- Choose somewhere comfortable to lie or sit. Make sure you are warm and will not be disturbed. You will need to allow at least 45 minutes. Light a candle and dedicate it to your journey and your joint experiences. Wrap yourself in a favourite blanket.

- Close your eyes and go within, inside to that place which is uniquely you. Bring your attention to your breath. Allow your breathing to be deep and gentle. Feel yourself becoming calm and relaxed.

- Link your physical body to your breathing by becoming aware of the gentle movement of your body in time with your breathing. Enjoy feeling this link and enjoy your body breathing on your behalf.

- Become aware of the rise and fall of energy entering and leaving your body. Allow yourself to ride these energy waves as you gather energy for your journey on the in-breath and allow your physical body and mind to let go on the out-breath. You are ready to begin exploring the next stage of your journey.

- You are going to die. There is nothing you can do to avoid this. Your death is definite. Stay with this truth for a few moments. Allow any thoughts and feelings this generates to be present. Be the observer to your human reaction to this truth.

- Allow an image to appear of a place where you would like to die. This can be anywhere – a place in nature, a favourite room. Spend a few minutes exploring this image, noticing any details. Is there anything you would like to have with you at the time of your death? Add it to your image. Allow yourself to be with the place of your death.

- As your death approaches you are reminded of some of the adventures you have experienced in your life. Allow any images of these adventures to appear. Be the observer, just as if you are watching a video.

- Your death draws closer. You have met with many people on your life path, some of whom have been very important to you. Allow some of these people to visit you now as you await your death. There may be some unfinished business. People may want to say goodbye. Spend time with these people.

- Death is near. You have given much of yourself to your life through the time and energy you have devoted to your work, to gathering material things about you. These have all contributed in part to your identity. Allow yourself to be reminded of what you have devoted your life energy to. Be the observer.

- Your death is only a breath away. Allow yourself to let go of your life experiences, the people you have met, your work, your material possesions, your identity. Breathe them away. Let go of life.

- Your death is now. Let go into death. Feel yourself opening up to the light of death. Allow the light of death to release you from your physical body, from your physical life.

- Allow yourself to be gently held in the light of death. Be with the light. Experience the light. Become the light. Experience the sense of freedom and spaciousness.

- Your death is complete. You are Light. Experience the joy of this new way of being. YOU ARE. You are Light. You are Joy. You are Peace. You are Love. Experience you. You are at one. YOU ARE. And now for the next stage of your journey.

- From somewhere comes the sound of a gently beating drum. Allow yourself to be drawn towards the sound. You are choosing to return to planet Earth. The journey is gentle.

- You are bringing the light with you. The drum beat grows louder.

- You are Light, you are Peace, you are Love. You are journeying, drawn by the sound of the drum. Your mother's heartbeat calls out to you. You respond – I am here. I am.

- It is dark. You are safe. You have everything you need. You are journeying. There is little room in this place. The drum beat grows louder and faster. Feel yourself responding to the call of the drum. There are many drums calling you.

- Move towards the light. Experience yourself leaving the womb. You are journeying. Feel yourself emerging into the world. You are journeying. There are many hearts beating, announcing your decision to join the Earth family. You have arrived safely. YOU ARE.

- Spend a few moments with this vision of arrival back on Earth. Allow your-self to just be.

- Bring your attention to your breathing. With every breath, feel yourself returning gently to a normal wakened state. Gradually become aware of your body and your blanket. Use your breathing to help you to connect fully with your body and with your surroundings.

- Open your eyes and spend a few moments relating to your surroundings. It may feel appropriate for your partner to hold your hand or to hold you.

- When you feel ready, share your experience with your partner. When there has been time for this, allow your partner to share their experiences of wit-nessing your journey with you.

(**Note:** *You should not switch roles in this exercise without allowing time for the experiences to be fully absorbed. The time needed will vary from person to person. We suggest a period of at least one month to elapse before witnessing your partner's journey.)*

By meditating on our own death and rebirth, we are constantly reviewing them and asking ourselves, what would make my life more meaningful, what could make my death more meaningful?

LEARNING ABOUT DYING

In her healing sessions, Julia discovered that dying was not something she was going to have to do, but something she was going to be. She learned how to be soul. The process of dying was leaving the physical body and being who she was – soul. And in this being she discovered that there was more Love, more Peace and more Light than she could have imagined when she was in her body. The discovery that there would always be enough love, brought great peace and through her entry into the peace she became aware that there would always be enough light. These discoveries confirmed what had been in Julia's heart, that death was the gateway to profound beauty and a cause for celebration.

To work with the light, to create love and peace, you need to experience for yourself that these things are unlimited and unconditional. It is possible for the healer who is working with the soul-based approach to help another person discover how to die because soul will be the teacher. But you will need to have addressed your own fears, anxieties and prejudices, and to have healed any feelings of grief, around the whole area of death, for soul to have the freedom to do this.

DEATH IS LINKING WITH SOUL

In every healing situation, the healer works to achieve that linking with soul, which comes in moments of being centred. This moment may occur when the person considers their own death. Like Julia, a patient can come to have a new attitude to death as each healing session brings them closer to soul, in preparation for the ultimate union (in what we call death).

The healer links the patient to the soul (thus completing the third side of the Healing Triangle) and facilitates the union so that decisions can be made about death. Preparation for death means looking at the quality of your life.

Not all deaths are planned or peaceful like the one described. Death may be a quick event or it may take time for a person to die. In cases of sudden death and death by accident or violence, the healer can send distant healing to help the person pass over and to address the mental and emotional shock of becoming disembodied without warning.

Many healers find that working with the dying becomes part of their practice. When this is the case, our attitudes need to be clear. We are there first of all to support the dying person and to offer help on an unconditional basis. Secondly, we are there to support those around the dying person, again on an unconditional basis.

FEELINGS ABOUT DEATH

If this is your work you need to understand how a terminally ill person may be feeling. Initially they may be in a state of shock or numbness, in denial or isolation. They may or may not be expressing their emotions. If they are expressing them, they could be as various forms of fear – panic, anxiety or anger. Emotions can also take the form of guilt or hostility and resentment. Along with depression there may be physical symptoms of distress. The terminally ill person may need to experience some or all of these feelings before they can accept their condition. With this may be a return to hope or faith.

There is no defined pattern of behaviour for anyone going through such experiences and the healer may be invited to enter the story at any stage. But your presence itself is healing when it is the same presence that you offer to any patient – accepting, respecting, non-judgemental and supportive – loving. The patient needs to know that your reason for being there is not based on pity, self-importance or self-interest. You do not have to like the condition, but you cannot fear it.

When a person has been weakened by illness and their own feelings around it, especially over a long period, healing provides the much needed energy that the patient needs to die with dignity.

THE PROCESS OF DEATH

Experience in the body ceases when soul has completed its mission. It is soul's impulse that decides the moment when we detach from the physical body and pass back to the subtle realms of being in the astral body. The etheric energy system, on which the physical body depended, becomes depolarized and is gradually withdrawn so that the life force no longer reaches the cells. Each nucleus gives its last instruction, which is to begin the process of disintegration and return the chemical components of the body to the Earth. But the life that animated the body has simply moved on into another form.

When we do return to the light, however long or short our stay here, we do not just remain in the memories of loved ones and friends. We leave an energy trace that continues to vibrate within the landscape and all those places we have touched. This is our gift to the Earth and all who inhabit her. Every energy trace influences the energy pattern of all that is and we can be aware of this through the network of consciousness.

WORKING WITH THE BEREAVED

Andrew was grief stricken. His wife of six months had been killed in a car accident the year before. He was receiving counselling but concerned friends suggested that he should try healing to help recover his will to live.

Over many sessions Andrew released the pain of losing his wife. Still very much in love, he couldn't face the prospect of life without her. Life was cruel, there was no God, he just wanted to die – to be with her.

Eventually he learned to relax and during a healing session he slipped into a healing dream. The energy scan revealed that he needed healing for the base and heart centres. This situation is typical in cases of bereavement where the person feels that their own survival (base centre) is threatened by the death or loss of a loved one (heart centre).

Later, an emotional Andrew told how, in the healing sleep, he had seen himself walking alone along a beach that had been a favourite with his wife. She had been a teacher and he described how they had spent many summer evenings walking along the shoreline together, with Lynne collecting shells and different coloured stones for her class to enjoy. 'But why should I see that?' he asked. I suggested that the image might have a healing element to it.

He dismissed this angrily. It was his mind torturing him with painful memories. 'Healing can't help me,' he shouted. 'And I will not be coming back!'

But two weeks later Andrew made another appointment. 'Something weird is going on. I've had two dreams where I'm back on that beach again.' With encouragement, Andrew relaxed, his breathing telling me that he was slipping into a healing sleep. His heart and base centres were still calling for healing energy.

On his return, he told how he saw himself walking alone on the same beach and watched as the figure bent down to pick up something, then turned, offering an outstretched hand. The hand opened to reveal a small, pink, heart-shaped stone. Andrew took the stone. 'I had it right here!' he said excitedly. 'It's a present from Lynne, I know it is.'

Andrew continued to come for healing for the next six months. One day he announced it would be his last session. He had made a trip to the beach. Smiling, he opened his hand and there was the pink, heart-shaped stone.

Two years later an excited Andrew telephoned to say that he was getting married. He had a new job and was intending to settle in America with his new wife. 'Oh, by the way – we met on a beach!'

You, the healer, may enter the story to work with the bereaved to find that the one left behind has the same range of feelings as the terminally ill person. The energy that rushes to and from the heart centre at these times accounts for what we call grief. All the centres are involved in grief, but it is the endeavour of the heart centre to bring balance to the system. This is more difficult when we love or feel attachment for the one who has died, for it places an extra energetic burden on the heart centre. In healing terms, in all situations where there is grief, the link centre of the base is also involved in supporting the heart and its efforts.

THE TASKS OF MOURNING

Soul's message to us, via the heart centre, is to become totally involved in our feelings and to set about the tasks of mourning – that is to work with the grief. The first task is to accept the reality of the loss. Andrew was certainly feeling the reality of his wife's death, but he could not accept it. His way of coping was to deny meaning, deny the spiritual in his life and to want to die himself. These feelings were preventing him from carrying out the second task of addressing the pain of his grief. During the healing sessions, he began to do this. And in the middle of them his soul found a way of helping him to move to the third task of mourning – to find ways of adjusting to a life where Lynne was no longer there.

As you can gather from Andrew's story, healing has a powerful role to play in helping a person totally engage with their grief and to mourn. This is the healthy, life-affirming way that we humans have evolved to deal with all the energies generated within us by loss. The way that we achieve the first three tasks of mourning will determine the outcome of the fourth task. This is often the most difficult, for it is about rediscovering our willingness to carry on with life. In Andrew's story, the healer's conviction about his patient's own healing potential was borne out by what happened in the healing sleep. His soul created a way of guiding him through his grief so that he emerged on the other side of mourning as a whole person who was able to celebrate life. His soul's way was to teach him about the continuity of love and that his own love was not a punishment but a gift.

Each Loss Reminds Us Of Our Other Losses

When the death of a loved one hits us, we are reminded of all the 'deaths' that we have had to go through in life. As we consider each of these deaths, we realize that they were the loss of something or some aspect of ourselves. All our losses are like little deaths and, if we have not processed all our feelings about those other deaths, the grief may suddenly be released.

As healers we need to reflect on the pattern of losses in our own life, so that we can understand the meaning of loss for those with whom we might be working. In doing so we might gain insight into the deep meaning of loss and why it has always been a fact of life.

If we could hover above even a small village we would see the multitude of losses that people are experiencing. A man is sitting in a doctor's waiting room because he is suffering from depression and has attempted suicide. He has been made redundant, lost his job. But with that loss he has lost his way of life, his workmates, his wage packet, his self esteem and his joy of living.

A mother is taking her child to school for the first time. He will lose her constant presence and a way of life in which he was the centre of attention. No wonder he cries. She must give up her child to the school and her life will never be the same again. No wonder she cries at the school gates.

Down the road, the post brings the envelope a man has been waiting for – his final divorce papers. But as he looks at them the realization sweeps over him that he has lost his wife, his marriage and a way of life.

Next door a young woman sits in an empty nursery, holding a small dress to her lips. Last week she had a miscarriage. After months of thinking about birth, she is left going over and over the death of her unborn child.

We need go no further. There is no one, it seems, who is shielded from loss.

LOSS AS A FEATURE OF CHANGE

At each phase of grief and at each task of mourning, the healer has a role to play in being with the person, while they move through a phase, move on to the next phase or move out of grief into new life. As we can see from Andrew's story, this does not mean we must forget in order to move on, in order to live. To live creatively, like the Oneness that we are, we have to accept that the actual process of creativity is a process of change. But when faced with change we can easily become less than who we really are.

When a favourite character in a TV soap is killed off, many viewers find they have to come to terms with feelings of loss. When a famous fizzy drink company wanted to change the characteristic shape of its bottles, there was such a public outcry that the company had to restore the old style or lose its sales. Change means loss and change challenges us to find the resources to cope.

We are often surprised and even angry at change. Yet the one constant ingredient of life is change. Once we can accept this, we have dealt with the energy-generating loss factor. Until then, we will behave like the bereaved and will ultimately have to address the four tasks of mourning – to accept the reality of the loss, to address the pain of grief, to adjust to a life where who or what was lost is no longer there, to carry on with life.

THE LESSONS OF LOSS

When an event challenges our beliefs, as it may do in times of great trauma, we can experience a loss of self and our world. In the depths of our distress, we find out what we believe, what we consider to be our world, who we consider we truly are.

A Jewish woman described how she had a great teaching about loss during her last year in the Auschwitz concentration camp. In an interview, 50 years later, Esther said, 'One day I said to myself, "They've taken away my parents, my brother, my family. They've taken away my clothes. They've taken away my possessions. They've taken away my home. They have taken away everything I have grown to love. But they can't take away my soul." And I vowed that they would not take away my soul. From that moment, I began to fight back!'

269

Esther realized that loss has an important function in our lives. Only when we lose something do we unleash the powerful force for self-discovery that is loss. We may come to realize too that loss is soul's way of asking, Who are you? And that soul is helping us to ask ourselves, Who am I?

Loss, then, is also a sacred ritual of the birth/death cycle that nourishes our process of growth and transformation. Here again, the two energy centres involved tend to be the heart and the base.

Take time with the next Action Point to work with soul in this way.

ACTION POINT 53 The Teachings of Loss

Developmental tool – identifying the energies of limitation and liberation that teach us about our true identity.

This exercise may also be used for self-healing.

You need to be relaxed and in a comfortable place where you will not be disturbed for an hour. Work through each part of the exercise carefully and honestly, making notes before moving on to the next question. Notice how you feel; your emotional and mental reactions.

- If you lose your money, who are you?

- If you lose your job, who are you?

- If you lose your home, who are you?

- If you lose a loved one, who are you?

- If you lose your friend, who are you?

- If you lose your reputation, who are you?

- If you lose your health, who are you?

- If you lose your life, who are you?

- Did you find you? If so, how did you know it was you?

You may need to visit parts of the exercise a few times to get your answer.
Now relax and focus on your heart centre. Breathe a few times into your heart centre. Work with the next part of the exercise, giving yourself the time and space to feel the impact of each question. Wait patiently for the still small voice of your soul to answer. Try not to assume what the answer will be.

- You have lost your money, who are you?

- You have lost your job, who are you?

- You have lost your home, who are you?

- You have lost a loved one, who are you?

- You have lost your friend, who are you?

- You have lost your reputation, who are you?

- You have lost your health, who are you?

- You are about to lose your life, who are you?

- Did you find you? Was it the same you? How will you recognize you from now on?

UNFINISHED BUSINESS

As Julia confronted her own death, she came to understand that in order to pass peacefully on to the next phase of her soul journey, she would have to be at peace with herself and with others. This meant reviewing her feelings about other people and her relationships to see if she felt at peace with them. Where there was no feeling of peace, she came across 'unfinished business' – someone needing forgiveness, a quarrel that needed mending, unspoken words needing to be said at last, telling someone she loved them, and so on.

271

She would conclude the business of her life and bring peace to others as well as herself in the process. This would 'wipe the slate clean', so that everyone concerned, including herself, could start afresh. She saw that having a courageous heart actually led to rebirth so that she could look forward to her own rebirth back into the world she had come from.

Of course it is not the healer's place to suggest what a person may have left unfinished in their life, nor to advise on who or what needs to be forgiven. But the healer's presence and their ability to access soul-guidance can act as the catalyst that helps the patient to consider peace as another form of love or light or Oneness. Dealing with such aspects of the troubled conscience or the troubled mind, which make themselves known during Sacred Mindfulness practice, is a requirement for communion with the deep silence of the soul.

A New Relationship With Death And Those Who Have Passed

Julia had the courage and the love to remember those close to her whom she would be leaving behind. When the healer is able to allow others to be present, while the patient is learning how to leave their body with grace, these others in turn learn about the process. They too experience the deep peace and love present and they are able to gain a new perspective on death and perhaps new feelings about their own passing.

Julia and her family learned about the continuity of life through direct experience during the healing sessions. She was thus able to assure her husband and family that the link of love between them could not be broken and that she would maintain it. What they learned in the weeks and months after her death was that a totally new relationship with Julia had been born, where they were still on the physical level and she was on a subtle/spiritual one. Once people can accept this, that the soul lives on, they can learn to keep the link of love alive until they too join the loved one.

Someone Who Loves You Is There To Meet You

As Julia made her final journey out of her physical body, she managed to tell

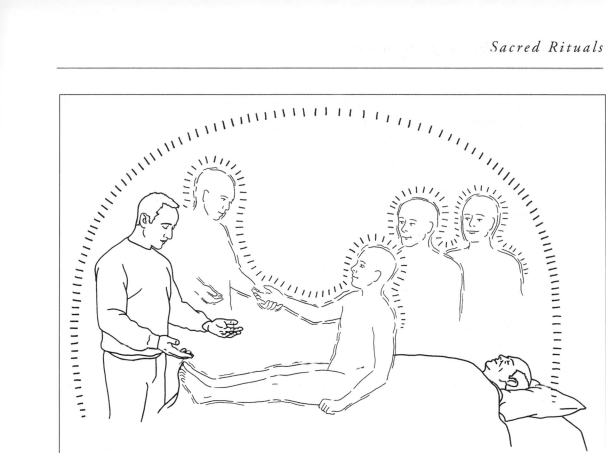

Figure 54. Passing over. The healer creates an energetic environment where the patient is helped to pass over. The deceased person sits up in his astral body. A loved one in spirit has come to greet him. Other spirit helpers stand close by.

the family that her mother (in spirit) had come to meet her. That there is always someone who loves you to greet you as you pass over has been confirmed many times. Nursing staff working with the terminally ill have told us how patients seemed to be talking to themselves, but when they paid closer attention to this they realized that the patients were talking to loved ones in spirit who had come to help them get used to leaving their bodies behind and to assure them that they would be there when the time came.

THE UNITY OF DEATH AND BIRTH

Through learning about the process of death experientially, we can understand that every death is also a birth. Death and birth are a unity, which perfectly illustrates the divine dichotomy of physical existence. For the unity is apparently two extremes.

But, like a coin, which can never be only one side or the other, human experience is that both birth and death are parts of a beautiful whole. All the little deaths that Esther died became rebirths for her. However, it is not the place of the healer, working with someone in the state of loss, to assure them that their loss is really a gain. The healer's role is to support such a person, just as they would in any other healing situation, knowing that soul will find a way of bringing them the information they need, the confirmation, the peace and light at the proper time.

You, as a healer, carer or therapist have had your cycle of births and deaths. Not one part of your life has been a mistake or happened in vain. The cycle has brought you to where you are now. Bless it and congratulate yourself that you have these experiences in your heart, which provide the base for your understanding of and compassion for others.

THE SYMBOLOGY OF BIRTH AND DEATH

Patients' stories show that there is always a choice about birth and death (beginning and ending), which needs to be made. For example, a person dreads the 'death' of what they know best, even though it is making them unwell. But they are not in the mental or emotional state where they can see that letting go would lead to birth into a new, more harmonious life. The body is their friend and soul will try to help them so that, sooner or later, the signal may be that unwell becomes illness. Finally, the illness forces that person to address what they needed to release – the wrong relationship, the wrong job, the unsuitable environment, etc.

Similarly, sickness can force whole families and communities to stop and reconsider the direction of their lives.

The planet, too, is constantly sending us messages about birth and death. Where illness may be seen as a disaster in someone's life, the planet is either being subjected to man-made disasters or it creates what seems like a disaster to us in the process of restoring planetary balance.

Through the symbology of births and deaths, human illness and planetary change show us that a death may need to happen before a rebirth can take place. The healing process may need destruction before regeneration. Illness may not be something to dread because it could be the prelude to a richer life. The patient may join this cycle and come for healing at any stage between breakdown and breakthrough.

HEALING AND BIRTH

You are part of the cycle of life, so find out all you can about the facts surrounding your own conception, time in the uterus and birth.

Many pregnant women come for healing, not because they or the foetus are unwell, but simply because they know about the benefits to both of them that a healing session will bring.

Most women are under a range of stresses and pressures. The unborn baby is part of the mother's system, and part of her emotional and mental life. Stress on the mother means some kind of stress, and so imbalance, for the baby. Healing offers both mother and baby the chance to restore harmony and this will also have a beneficial effect on the father and those others with whom the mother comes into contact.

In the next case study, we show how, if Daniella had known about healing when she was giving birth, she would have avoided years of unnecessary pain.

Daniella decided to seek healing for intense leg pain. There was nothing obviously wrong with her upper legs or her lower back and her doctor had prescribed pain-killers. Her story focused on the pain and she expressed bewilderment as to its origin.

The scan of the energy circuits revealed a break in the middle of the pelvis and at the base of the spine. This was affecting the energies of both legs.

As healing energy was directed to the pelvic area and the base of the spine, Daniella said, 'I had a bad experience with Marco's birth. It was very long and ended with a forceps delivery. I felt extremely bruised for months after. But that was 11 years ago.'

The healing was encouraging her to connect her current pain with a past experience. Daniella's base centre was also affected by the difficult birth. Meanwhile, she had lived with the damaged energy circuits. Since then she had often experienced pain at the base of the spine or in her legs.

It took a few sessions to repair the circuit damage, but after each session Daniella's pain diminished until it disappeared and did not return.

It came as no surprise when Daniella spoke of a much improved relationship with her son, Marco. Healing had helped Daniella and restored the bond between mother and son.

Under UK law, healers are not allowed to attend the mother until ten days after the birth, but Daniella's story points out the vast amount of work that can be done once this time has elapsed.

Even during the ten-day period, there is nothing to stop you from sending distant healing to a mother and/or her baby if this has been requested.

UNDERSTANDING SOUL'S PURPOSE

What a challenge it would be for parents, doctors and teachers to try to understand soul's purpose. And if they knew soul's purpose, how different their attitudes might be to the experiences surrounding birth and death.

When we see the newborn child, we are tempted by its tiny size to imagine it as a tiny soul. The soul has no 'size', but it would be far more helpful for us to realize the trauma of the soul's descent into a tiny, restricting and confining body.

There is always distress around a miscarriage, the death of a baby or the birth of a child with a defect or life-threatening condition. Much of this distress is due to our attitude towards these things. The soul cannot be hurt or injured. The soul chooses its life and the length of its life. It may or may not choose to experience birth. These teachings should never be thrust on to distressed parents, but if asked you can state the knowledge and experience of Sacred Healing. We urge people to honour the soul and the soul's needs, and to open their hearts to the possibility that we can commune with the soul of any baby or child.

All the above applies to any adult person who may be very ill or who seems to us to have died in a way that makes no sense to those of us who are left behind. Our minds may never give us satisfactory answers about birth, life and death, but it is certain that soul will. All we have to do is to have the respect to take the time to listen in our hearts for the voice of soul.

Meanwhile, it is the job of healing to support any person in time of need, realizing that not one being is separate from another.

Working with this handbook may well be a 'birth' for you. With the insights you have gained so far, you may be able to look at Mary's story (Chapter 3, The Soul Journey) again with new 'eyes'.

As you near the end of your journey through the book, we place life experience within the context of home to ask ourselves whether Spiritual Healing has any role to play in the fundamental gathering of human life we call community.

18

Sacred Community

In this last chapter we come full circle, from the sacred meeting place of a desert community in America to the sacred healing dance of a desert community in Africa. It is a dance that has evolved from many centuries of celebrating life and spirituality, and the elements of its healing power contain all that is needed to create sacred community.

The central event in the healing tradition of the Ju-hoansi people of the Kalahari desert, is the healing dance. This lasts all night, taking place four or five times a month and involves everyone in the camp. After sundown, some of the women sit around the fire singing and clapping a rhythm that signals the start of the healing dance. Soon they are joined by the men and other women, including the healers, who begin to dance around the singers.

As the dance becomes more intense, the healers experience spiritual energy moving up the spine. When this reaches the brow and crown centres the healers describe the state as 'thinking nothing'. They enter a state of enhanced awareness or transcendence, which is not a trance, but where they can travel in their astral bodies to heal others, even at a great distance. The women sense when the transcendent state has arrived and rise up on their knees as a feeling of great joy fills their hearts. 'We do this when our hearts are happy,' they say.

The Ju-hoansi people consider that healing involves health and growth on all levels, affecting the individual, the community, the environment and the entire cosmos. Their world-view makes no distinction between their physical, emotional and spiritual needs. Arguments, disagreements and psychological problems are wounds in the body of the whole group and not just those involved.

But although the healing dance is their main method of treating illness, this is not its prime function. The deeper purpose of the healing dance is to provide an opportunity for the people to join together in a spiritual journey during which the whole community is healed and reintegrated. What did not serve the community is allowed to die so that each member can be reborn.

Many so-called underdeveloped societies still have ceremonial ways that offer the community as a whole an opportunity to express and integrate its shadow aspect and to heal any conditions the shadow has created. In Bali, in Asia, for example, there is a dramatic ritual to disperse the tensions and bad feelings that have accumulated in a village. These are embodied in the part of the 'demon' and the dispersal of negativity is carried out by its clash with the 'warrior'. This is the famous *Ketchak* dance. Here, the men dance in concentric circles into which the communal village demon enters, to be overthrown by the hero warrior. After offerings to the gods and spirits have been made, the healing of the village is complete.

All societies need a way to heal communal malaise if they are to remain healthy. The more industrialized societies tend to demonize their shadow aspects to make individuals or groups the scapegoats who can then be the focus of public scorn, disgust and even violence. The healing of the community, however, has not taken place and the fear remains to take the form of further scapegoating.

While the healing dance is still a spiritual focus for many indigenous communities, people in the west are seeking a new spiritual focus as they see the process of technological change undermining what they considered were their spiritual values. Many are wondering what those values were and whether established religion ever was the guardian and nurturer of our spirituality.

In the field of health care, many disciplines are debating what the role of the spiritual might mean for them or how this dimension could be incorporated into their work.

The spiritual dimension is already the core of our work, but we feel that the healing dance challenges healers to ask themselves, What is my purpose in the community in which I find myself?

The Lakota healer, Frank Fools Crow, whom we mentioned in Chapter 4, The New Healer, had a very clear idea of why the healer archetype exists at all in any community. For him, healing an individual only had value in terms of what it teaches the people. 'Seeing a person healed is confirmation to the community that God is with them,' he said.

Spiritual Healing holds the view that the role for healers is the same as the healing dance, where a channel is created for the inflow of spiritual power into the community. As this is demonstrated through the healing of people, situations and the environment, the community receives confirmation that 'God is with them'. This is what sustains any community, giving it the strength and assurance to carry on in the face of any distress or disaster.

For western societies it would bring soul from its current place at the margins, to its desperately needed place at the centre of the community. This does not mean that healers are replacing the function of religion, but it does mean that they are playing their part in the respiritualization of all aspects of human life, for which the people of the world are calling.

HEALING PRACTICE AS HEALING DANCE

To give us some idea of how healing practice could become a healing dance, let's look at the dance to see what aspects create the basis of sacred community. We have identified the following:

- **Being in communion.** The people commune together and act together for a sacred purpose.
- **Inviting in soul.** The people create ceremony and celebrate life and the presence of the spiritual in life.
- **The spiritual perspective and world-view is founded on the Oneness of all that is.** This means that what affects one affects all.

- **Arousal of spiritual energy.** The state of 'no thought' is the healing state. This activates astral healing.
- **Astral travel.** The healers leave their physical body to travel to help others.
- **The people journey together.** The dance is a special form of communal journeying towards reintegration and rebirth.
- **Letting go.** The people are able to let go of what no longer serves them. In so doing they heal others and the cosmos.
- **Healing energy is sensed as joy.** The people recognize the creative nature of healing energy.
- **Polarity balance.** The 'feminine' polarity of the healing dance's energy is a receptacle for creative healing joy. The women of the group act out this role. The 'masculine' polarity is the active delivery of the energy. The men of the group act out this role.

Now let's see if there are any parallels with the practice of Spiritual Healing.

Communion

Your Sacred Mindfulness practice is communion with soul. This could be done on a regular basis with small or large groups, where communion is also with each soul and with the group energy.

Inviting soul in

Attunement invites soul in and this is reinforced by the attitude of asking soul to guide the healing, via the intuitive approach to the work. We saw in the distant healing circle how a simple ceremony can bind people together to provide the beginnings of healing celebration. But there is a place here for more ceremony and more celebration.

Ceremony is central to the life of the heart and the sacred community. We make ourselves available to soul and invite soul in to be expressed through the ceremony and on into the life of the community. We can do ceremony on our own or with others. When we do it together, like the healing dance, it reminds us that we are part of one another and that we are together in Oneness. Ceremony is one of soul's ways of having a party and the best parties are with other people.

It is the healer's business to do all this, so ritual and ceremony may well become part of your practice, as it did for Dr Mehl-Madrona (see *Coyote Medicine* in Further Reading). He found that his practice as a highly qualified physician in the US was greatly enhanced when he incorporated ritual and ceremony into his work. Each healing ceremony was created with the patient for a specific purpose at a particular time in the treatment.

World-view

The perspective of Spiritual Healing is clear. The healer's respect and unconditional positive regard for the patient is based on their inner knowledge that no person or being is separate from any other. This practice attitude must be extended to those with whom we do not work and further into the wider community and the world.

The best example is one who acts on the basis of the Spiritual Healing world-view. This is beautifully expressed in the Lakota declaration of Oneness: *Mitakuye oyasin! – we are all related* or *all my relations* – which is used in all Lakota sacred ceremonies. You will recall that the healer and holy man, Fools Crow, belonged to this Native American Nation.

Arousal of spiritual energy

The state of 'no thought' in the dancing healers is similar to the ideal working mode of the healer. The same state may be achieved in deep meditation.

But when this happens as a result of the arousal of spiritual energy (*kundalini*) outside a situation like the healing dance, some people fear its effects. We have counselled against forcing this process (see Chapter 8, Seven Sacred Steps), but when it is aroused unintentionally by a gentle practice such as a meditation or group visualization, this has only happened because the time is right for that person. Instead of fearing any distress that arousal might cause, the person should relax and allow things to take their course. Healers can be supportive at such times if they too have no fear and consciously retain their healing presence.

Astral travel

We described in Chapter 16, Distant Healing, how this can be a special part of healing work. It is a natural outcome of attaining the 'no thought' or deep meditation state. Healers could use astral travelling when intuitively inspired to look elsewhere in the community to see who or what needs help.

Journeying together

The healer and the patient set out on a spiritual journey when they agree to work together.

Most of our work with groups has involved such a journey and group members have shown how they are looking for sacred community within the workshop situation.

The concept of the mutual journey in other relationships is an actuality of which we are generally unconscious. The healer can make this their conscious choice.

Letting go

The patient is encouraged, through the opening up and rebalancing of the subtle energy system, to let go of what no longer allows them to express and to be who they really are.

The healer needs to have the same experience through addressing their own personal transformation. Remember, you are offering the patient your own energy field, your hollow bone. Letting go clears and harmonizes the field and strengthens the healing channel.

Healing energy is joy

Joy, and joy at the recovery of peace, are often the expression of healing in a patient. Joy is a healing energy because it is creative, emanating as it does from the sacral centre. The healer must be well acquainted with joy and creativity in their own life, and look for ways to bring this into the community.

Ask yourself when you last experienced healing energy (not a cure or patient gratitude) as pure joy? This can be something to be alert for in the future. Joy in any situation is a sign that healing is taking place on some level.

Polarity balance

As the healing procedure described in Chapter 14 shows, healers work very carefully with polarity balance. We also need to look at ourselves to see if our own patterns are balanced. Our receptive/'feminine' energies need to be in harmony with our giving/'masculine' energies. We have the power to choose how we use these energies and for healers they must be in balance.

Within any community there is a second energy polarity with which the New Healer can deal. This is the polarity of energetic compatibility and incompatibility – who or what does or does not resonate with us.

Through developing heightened awareness, the healer is able to be aware of and understand what happens in similar and dissimilar energetic relationships. When we are aware of the energy of a situation or a person, we can begin to identify how it differs or is incompatible with our own.

This alertness allows us to respond to energetic situations that may cause problems in our relationships, which would, in turn, create heavy energy. Similarly, awareness helps us to discover areas of compatibility from which we can begin to harmonize the energies to empower all parties.

In all relationships where the energies are dissimilar to our own, the technique is to clear the energy field, if it has accumulated heavy energy (as in Action Point 8), rather than to try to change the relationship. Harmony is not the same as balance, but an energetic state of tolerance and mutually constructive compromise, where the aim is not for each party to be the same, but for each to agree to be different and to tolerate the difference. This can lead to everyone being able to honour and celebrate their differences, which is harmony.

By consciously developing energetic harmony, we ensure that we maintain well-being and a flexibility that allows us to embrace and flow through all situations of unpredictability and uncertainty. With this approach we can recognize such situations as creative possibilities. Practice with this energetic polarity (tolerance) will soon show you the beneficial effects.

MEETING THE NEEDS OF OUR NEW ROLE

There do seem, then, to be many parallels between Spiritual Healing and the healing dance. But if our intention is to make our practice a catalyst for creating sacred community, this has to be a conscious and responsible decision.

Individual healers, through their procedures and attunement, are inviting soul into those places where they operate – wherever they might be. This creates centres of light that radiate out into the wider world, encouraging new types of community to take root and grow.

We have provided the channel for the impact of spiritual energy into the community and we have set up energetic fields for which we are now responsible. Are we ready as healers and as people for the responsibility of creating new communities – for this is what we are doing? Do we have everything in place in terms of meeting the needs of our new role as channels for the power of soul into the community?

For guidance in how to meet these needs, we refer again to the Seven Places of Peace in Chapter 5. The community needs us to combine them with those practices and procedures that parallel the healing dance.

Peace is not the absence of strife but the presence of soul. When the people walk in peace, they walk with soul, they look to bring harmony, they 'walk in Beauty', as the Navajo say.

To walk in Beauty the community needs us to have faith in life and in soul, and to celebrate both. Our healing needs to show the people that there is enough for all our needs. There is enough love and healers make this love available. This is the foundation of healing.

The community needs us to open our hearts to one another and exchange love. This is the first step towards a renewal of the community so our healing presence must be whole-hearted.

The community needs us to shine, to bring laughter. We need to be absolutely serious in our pursuit of lightness and non-judgemental in all our dealings with patients and the people.

The community needs us to be intuitively aware so that we are aware of and sensitive to each other's needs, and to the needs of the planet and the Earth family. The basis of the healing procedure is this level of awareness, not the performance of a set routine.

The community needs us to honour life, the life force and the subtle realms of being and the part they play in healing.

The community needs us to live creatively, to make our healing a creative act. This will allow us to welcome the challenges of change.

The community needs us to be clear hollow bones, to have pure intention and to be authentic. Self-development is needed, along with healing experience as part of our spiritual life. Following personal transformation, we will need to look carefully at how we manage our environment, how we manage our organizations and how we manage the impact of the organizations on the environment. The community needs us to be an example of walking in Beauty – to bring Peace, Love and Light from the healing session into life and our dealings with the people.

THE NEW HEALER AND THE SACRED COMMUNITY

The New Healer understands how the needs of our time have changed the role of the healer. Each healing session must not only care for the individual, but also go to build those sacred communities, which will become the spiritual power points that are needed for the transformation of all structures of society.

Imagine how education, health care, economics, politics, foreign policy, etc. would change once the concept of Oneness became understood, acknowledged and accepted.

It is worth imagining a world where the loved-based approach to all problems would be treated as a priority.

The New Healer understands that healing is nothing less than the deep healing of the entire human family, the healing of the Earth and the Earth family. It can be done when each community becomes a place where soul is invited in. Then healing will be a celebration of life, of the journey of the soul and of being.

This is the vision of Spiritual Healing. It is up to us to 'ground' the vision.

NOW IT'S TIME TO CELEBRATE

We invite you to celebrate with a simple ceremony. First, think about your next step. At some point, by yourself or with your family or some friends, light a candle and dedicate the light to ... your next step ... your vision of sacred community ... your vision of sacred healing ... the recognition of Oneness ... Peace ... how you will ground your vision ...

Think of all the candles that will be lit, all the dances that will be danced, and how one day you will meet someone who has lit a candle to celebrate too.

Glossary

Astral: any level of being outside the physical. The astral body is the energy pattern used by soul to travel on these levels.

Aura: the total emanation of the human, including the physical, etheric, and other energy zones. The human energy field.

Avatar: a physical manifestation (usually human) of the Source whose role is to bring Love, Peace and Light to this level of existence. Sanskrit, *avatara*.

Centre: see energy centre.

Chakra: now a common term for a subtle energy centre. See energy centre. From Sanskrit, *chakram*, 'wheel'. The whirling vortex of energy looks somewhat like a turning wheel.

Contact healing: healing where the patient is present.

Distant healing: healing where the patient is at a distance from the healer. Includes astral level healing. Also known as absent healing (in the patient's absence).

Earth: planet Earth. In Spiritual Healing, the living organism which we inhabit, that has its own path of evolution and subtle levels.

Earth Family: all other beings, apart from humans, who inhabit the Earth (to distinguish them from humans), such as animals, plants, etc.

Emotional: the subtle energy zone in a person's energy field where emotional and feeling material is stored and/or processed.

Energy: in Spiritual Healing, a force directed by and emanating from the Source. Spirit is the energy of the Source. The physical has a relatively low frequency of energy.

Energy centre: a subtle structure, situated in the etheric body, designed to allow the flow of subtle energies into and out of the human body and energy field. See also, chakra.

Energy field: see aura.

Etheric: the level of being next to the physical at which energy vibrates at a higher frequency. The etheric body is the subtle communication vehicle of the soul and the support system for the physical body.

Field: short form of energy field, aura.

Holistic: in therapy, applied to the whole person, rather than a specific part or condition. The whole person at every level of their being and further, including the whole of creation.

Hollow bone: Fools Crow's term for the healer's ability to be a vehicle for healing energies. Such a person is also known as a 'hollow bone'.

Incarnation: birth on the Earth (physical) level of being. The taking on of a physical body for the soul (spirit) to experience this level.

Intuitive: inner knowing or sensing at a soul level which is transmitted by the brow centre to the solar plexus, via the heart centre. In Sacred Healing, the soul-based or soul-guided approach.

Kundalini: potential energy of spiritual illumination stored in the base centre. It activates, clears and aligns the energy centres. From Sanskrit, *Kundal*, a coil, and *ini*, the feminine ending.

Kirlian: in 1939, the Russians Semyon and Valentina Kirlian rediscovered 'corona discharge' photography which uses a high frequency electric discharge to 'photograph' the radiations from living material.

Level: a plane of being or experience where energy vibrates at a certain frequency according to the level. A stage of evolution. A state of consciousness.

Life force: the vital energy which is essential to life, conducted by the subtle energy system of the etheric body. Sanskrit, *prana*. Chinese *qi*. Japanese *ki*.

Light: an aspect of spiritual energy. A force which tends towards healing and enlightenment. When Light (with a capital letter), healing energy.

Love: an aspect of spiritual energy. A force which tends towards integration. When Love (with a capital letter) healing energy.

Mental: the subtle energy zone in a person's energy field where mental/thought material is stored and/or processed.

Oneness: a term describing the Source as all that is. Used by Australian Aboriginals to mean the same.

Out-of-body: the experience of being out of the physical body (travelling in the astral body), in which a person is not controlled by physical limitations. For all people, part of the experience of sleep.

Patient: in Spiritual Healing, a term to distinguish the person you are working with when healing. It does not denote that there is something wrong or that there is a problem.

Peace: an aspect of spiritual energy. A force of reciprocity and harmony. When Peace (with a capital letter), healing energy.

Personality: the physical consciousness of self that tends to see itself as separate from the Source/soul.

Psychic: a subtle sense, monitored by the brow centre, for detecting and sensing subtle energies and their manifestations. The way our brain interprets this information is our perception of it. Not to be confused with 'intuitive'. Everyone has intuitive and psychic senses at various stages of development and different people's perceptions of the same subtle phenomenon will vary.

Qi Gong: the Chinese system of exercises where breath and movement are used to enhance the intake and flow of *qi*, the life force.

Reincarnation: being born more than once on the Earth plane. The theory (borne out by worldwide research) which proposes this process as a natural part of the human soul journey because we tend not to remember, express and create who we really are in one lifetime (incarnation).

Sacred: pertaining to the spiritual in life. The spiritual aspect of any thing or person.

Sai Baba: acknowledged by millions of followers worldwide to be an *avatar*. He was born in India on 23 November 1926. He has prophesised that he will pass over in 2022 and reincarnate as Prema (Love) Sai Baba.

Soul: in this book: a spiritual and energetic reality - the incarnated human spirit. Our true nature. Since there is no actual separation between one soul and another, the word 'soul' (without an article such as 'the' or 'a') is also a term for the Source, Oneness, the God within.

Soul journey: your human life, seen in terms of the journeying soul. Or can be seen as a journey through many experiences, on many levels, some of which may be on planet Earth, or other parts of the universe.

Source: All That Is. All energy. In religious terms - God, the Creator. Oneness.

Spirit: the energy of the Source which can take any form. All life is spirit. When 'in spirit', denotes a person or being from a subtle level (not in a physical body).

Spiritual: in Spiritual Healing, all that is to do with soul, the spirit and the Source.

Spiritual Healing: a form of subtle energy medicine which has the soul-based, intuitive approach as its core strategy.

Spirituality: any spiritual activity which inclines you to the Source, soul, your true self. Also, a person's true self.

Subtle: energy vibrating at a higher frequency than the physical. Such energy, travelling at a velocity beyond the speed of light, behaves in very different ways to those physical energies known to most science. The 'fifth' force.

Subtle energy medicine: any therapy which works primarily with the subtle energy system to bring balance and/or harmony to the patient.

Subtle energy system: the co-ordinated system of the etheric body, comprising the energy centres and their etheric network links, and the other zones of the energy field.

Further Reading

Angelo, Jack, *Spiritual Healing: Energy Medicine for Health and Well-Being*, Element Books, Shaftesbury, 1991.

Angelo, Jack, *Your Healing Power*, Piatkus Books, London, 1994/98.

Angelo, Jack, *Hands-On Healing*, Healing Arts Press, Rochester, Vermont, 1997.

Assagioli, Roberto, *Psychosynthesis*, Aquarian Press, London & San Francisco, 1993.

Bailey, Alice, *Esoteric Healing*, Lucis Press, London & New York, 1993.

Bancroft, Anne, *Weavers of Wisdom: Women Mystics of the Twentieth Century*, Arkana/Penguin, London & New York, 1989.

Carey, Ken, *Flatrock Journal: A Day in the Ozark Mountains*, HarperCollins, New York, 1993.

Cousineau, Phil, ed. *The Hero's Journey: Joseph Campbell on his Life and Work*, HarperSanFrancisco, New York, 1991.

Gerber, Richard, *Vibrational Medicine*, Bear and Company, Santa Fe, NM, 1988/96.

Gerber, Richard, *Vibrational Medicine for the 21st Century*, Piatkus Books, London 2000.

Hunt, Valerie, *Infinite Mind: The Science of Human Vibrations*, Malibu Publishing, Malibu, CA, 1995.

Katz, Richard, Biesele, Megan and St Denis, Verna, *Healing Makes Our Hearts Happy: Spiritual Healing Among the Kalahari Ju-hoansi*, Inner Traditions, Rochester, Vermont, 1997.

Krippner, S. and Welch, P., *Spiritual Dimensions of Healing*, Irvington Publications, New York, 1992.

Kubler-Ross, Elisabeth, *On Death and Dying*, Macmillan, London & New York, 1970.

Mails, Thomas E., *Fools Crow: Wisdom and Power*, Council Oak Books, Tulsa, OK, 1991.

Mehl-Madrona, Lewis, *Coyote Medicine: Lessons From Native American Healing*, Scribner, New York/Rider, London 1997.

Moore, Thomas, *Care of the Soul*, HarperCollins, New York/Piatkus Books, London 1992.

Moore, Thomas, *The Re-Enchantment of Everyday Life*, Hodder & Stoughton, London, 1996.

Morgan, Marlo, *Mutant Message From Forever*, Thorsons, London, 2000.

Oschman, J.L., *Readings on the Scientific Basis of Bodywork, Movement and Energetic Therapies,* NORA Press, Dover, NH, 1997.

Rinpoche, Sogyal, *The Tibetan Book of Living and Dying*, Rider, London, 1992.

Rogers, Carl R., *A Way of Being*, Houghton Mifflin, New York, 1995.

Thorne, Brian, *Person-Centred Counselling*, Whurr, London & New Jersey, 1998.

Tiller, William A., *What Are Subtle Energies? Journal of Scientific Exploration*, Vol 7, No 3, 1993.

Trevelyan, George, *Magic Casements: The Use of Poetry in the Expanding of Consciousness*, Coventure, London, 1980.

Walsch, Neale Donald, *Communion With God*, Hodder & Stoughton, London, 2000.

Whitmore, Diana, *Psychosynthesis Counselling In Action*, Sage Publications, London & Newbury Park, CA, 1991.

Wilcox, Joan Parisi, *Keepers of the Ancient Knowledge: the Mystical World of the Q'ero Indians of Peru*, Element Books, London & Boston, MA, 1999.

Website Resources

Organizations concerned with subtle energy medicine, spiritual healing and related complementary therapies

British Alliance of Healing Associations
www.bahahealing.co.uk

British Complementary Medicine Association
www.bcma.org

College of Psychic Studies
www.collegeofpsychicstudies.co.uk

Confederation of Healing Organisations (UK)
www.confederation-of-healing-organisations.org

Association for Research and Enlightenment (US)
www.edgarcayce.org

International Society for Complementary Medicine Research (US)
www.iscmr.org

International Society for the Study of Subtle Energy and Energy Medicine (US)
www.issseem.org

Lucis Trust (UK)
www.lucistrust.org

National Federation of Spiritual Healing
www.nfsh.org.uk

Institute of Noetic Sciences (US)
www.noetic.org

Scientific and Medical Network (UK)
www.scimednet.org

Spiritualist Association of Great Britian
www.sagb.org.uk

Spiritualist National Union (UK)
www.snu.org

White Eagle Lodge (UK)
www.whiteagle.org

AUSTRALIA, CANADA, NEW ZEALAND, SOUTH AFRICA
There are a number of healing organizations in these countries that are affiliated to the NFSH (UK). For information contact the NFSH at their address above.

Journals carrying articles on spiritual healing and related topics

Caduceus (UK)
www.caduceus.info

Healing Today
(journal of the NFSH)

Journal of Alternative and Complementary Medicine
(journal of the International Society for Complementary Medicine Research)

Light
(journal of the College of Psychic Studies)

Living Lightly
(magazine form of *Positive News* –
www.positivenews.org.uk)

Resurgence (UK)
www.resurgence.org

Shift
(journal of the Institute of Noetic Sciences)

Subtle Energies and Energy Medicine
(journal of ISSSEEM)

Venture Inward
(journal of the Association for Research and Enlightenment)

Counselling, psychotherapy, transpersonal psychology and the person-centred approach
For details of courses, workshops and registered practitioners:

British Association for Counselling and Psychotherapy
www.bacp.co.uk

British Association for the Person-Centred Approach
www.bapca.org.uk

Psychosynthesis and Education Trust (UK)
www.psychosynthesis.edu

Institute of Psychosynthesis (UK)
www.psychosynthesis.org

Centre for Transpersonal Psychology
www.transpersonalcentre.co.uk

For counselling skills training: contact your local adult education/further education college. Many courses are offered in a variety of formats.

Index